D0810999

Doctors Talking

7 5 016

A 7 87 5

By the same author:

A Handbook of Sick Visiting
Making Use of Illness
Visiting the Sick
Learning about Christian
    Health and Healing
Learning about the Dying

CHICAGO PUBLIC LIBRARY

R00542 38134

Doctors Talking

A Guide to current Medico-Moral
Problems

by

Norman Autton

Chaplain, University Hospital of Wales, Cardiff

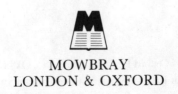

MOWBRAY
LONDON & OXFORD

Copyright © Norman Autton 1984

ISBN 0 264 66894 4

First published 1984
by A. R. Mowbray & Co. Ltd,
Saint Thomas House, Becket Street,
Oxford, OX1 1SJ

All rights reserved. No part of this publication
may be reproduced, stored in a retrieval system,
or transmitted, in any form or by any means,
electronic, mechanical, photocopying, recording,
or otherwise, without the prior permission in writing
from the publisher, A. R. Mowbray & Co. Ltd.

British Library Cataloguing in Publication Data

Autton, Norman
    Doctors talking.
    1. Medical ethics
    I. Title
    174'.2   R724

    ISBN 0–264–66894–4

Phototypeset by Oxford Publishing Services, Oxford
Printed in Great Britain by Spottiswoode Ballantyne Ltd, Colchester.

851
B

10.95

AD
KATIE
MICHAEL, SARA
MARY, RICHARD, JAYNE

OMNES AMATI BENE

Contents

Foreword by The Archbishop of York   *page*   ix

Preface   xi

Introduction   1

1. Human Experimentation   9

2. Organ Transplantation   47

3. Brain-Death   81

4. Handicapped Infants — To Live or Let Die?   108

5. Human Fertilization and Embryology   154

The Warnock Report   203

Appendix I: (a) Nuremberg Code   205

           (b) Declaration of Helsinki   207

Appendix II: Human Tissue Act 1961   210

Appendix III: Questions for Discussion   213

Glossary   216

References   220

Index of Proper Names   235

Index of Subjects   237

Foreword

The special quality of this book is apparent even from the title. Canon Autton, as the doyen of hospital chaplains, has had a lifetime's opportunity to listen to doctors talking. He has therefore been able to provide more than the reasoned and well-informed discussion of medico-moral problems which admirers of his previous books might have expected of him. By allowing doctors whenever possible to speak for themselves, he has managed to convey some of the nuances of actual decision-making.

Nuanced discussions of intractable ethical problems are hard to write, but of far more value to practitioners in this field than attempts to produce clear-cut but over-simple 'answers'. It is by standing alongside others who have wrestled with the problems, and by being drawn, as it were, into the conversation, that the best help can be found. I believe that this is what Canon Autton enables his readers, both lay and professional, to do, and that his book is a valuable addition to the literature on some painful human dilemmas.

Bishopthorpe, York † John Ebor:
30 April 1984

Preface

This is a book of many contributors, and without the goodwill and co-operation of a number of leading representatives in the field of medicine and ethics such a volume could not have been produced. For such collaboration and team-work I am extremely grateful.

I wish to express appreciation to both Mr Kenneth Baker and Canon William Purcell, respectively Managing Director, Publishing, and Literary Adviser to Messrs Mowbray, for granting me a 'roving commission' to visit various medical centres and research units throughout the country in order to discuss with surgeons, physicians and research workers some of the medico-moral issues which are at present of major concern to Church and Medicine. Permission was readily granted for talks and dialogues to be tape-recorded and relevant extracts to be interpolated into the text. Where time or distance made a personal encounter impractical a number of doctors readily responded to letters or questionnaires. All those who contributed and shared freely their viewpoints and opinions are officially acknowledged on pages 2–8.

One of the unhelpful features of some of the current debates on the topics under consideration is the tendency of a number of discussants to express clear-cut answers or reach absolutist conclusions without first having studied sufficiently the medical context or taken into account the full scientific facts. In order that the medical information outlined in the following chapters be as accurate and up-to-date as possible each has been read through and commented upon in its original draft by a leading authority in the respective field of study. While his comments have been much appreciated the official reader is in no way to be held responsible for the views expressed or the inadequacies displayed by the author.

It is my privilege to serve as chaplain to a very large and modern Medical Centre, and have official access to the Medical School library. To the librarians concerned I convey my sincere thanks for their readiness at all times to make available medical text-books, journals, and periodicals which it has been essential to study in pursuit of the medical background relevant to the subjects which comprise the chapters of this book.

My secretary, Mrs Anne Taylor, has not only been faced with the arduous task of typing the manuscript, but also the additional work of transcribing a large number of tape-recordings. I am personally much indebted to her for the very efficient and painstaking manner in which she has so cheerfully accomplished her two-fold task.

Finally I wish to record my gratitude to the medical and para-medical staff of the University Hospital of Wales for their friendship and encouragement. Such generous support has meant much in the undertaking of this study.

6 January 1984   Norman Autton
(*Feast of the Epiphany*)   Chaplain, University Hospital of Wales, Cardiff

Introduction

The role and function of a hospital chaplain is becoming more and more comprehensive and out-reaching; his opportunities are widening and his relationships with other members of staff more firmly established. It is vital that he works in a satisfactory relationship with the medical staff, for his ministry is complementary to that of the doctor as part of the total care of the patient. Such co-operative relationships are mutual, for all disciplines working harmoniously together contribute to and receive from each other the essential components for total health care.

In the sphere of medical ethics, while other disciplines *may* raise the kinds of ethical questions that are important to quality of treatment and recognition of human need, the hospital chaplain *must* raise these issues. It is that compulsion which should make chaplains more and more conscious of and sensitive to such problems and bring them to the fore in deliberation with members of various treatment teams both in hospital and in community.

As well as hospital ward and unit the debate concerns parish and parochial life, and it is the duty of the hospital chaplain to bring medical and ethical concerns to the notice of his colleagues in the community, so that in turn they themselves may initiate discussions and debates and so influence their people at large to think seriously and pray regularly about some of the important and tantalizing ethical problems not only confronting and challenging the world of Medicine but also the Church and its traditional teachings.

Technology is leaping ahead faster than the average layperson's understanding of its implications. While great care and judgement must be exercised in evaluating the contributions which modern scientific techniques can bring to a truly human life, it has to be recognized that no longer can the churchman turn to a traditional theology to help him solve some of our present medico-moral dilemmas, for many of

1

them are entirely new, little dreamt of by our forefathers in the faith. As much as he may long for them he will search in vain for 'answers' as such. It is this which makes the challenge so exciting and stimulating.

It is one thing to theorize about these problems in the neutral and comfortable environment of the lecture room or study; to pontificate and moralize in committee, or become certain about one's attitudes after reading an official report, but it is quite another to be involved personally at the sharp end of life and death decisions in the clinical setting of a busy hospital ward, operating theatre, or intensive care unit. It is for this very reason that dialogue, to become fruitful and productive, should involve those members of the medical profession who are actively engaged in and personally confronted by heart-searching questionings and agonizing enigmas.

What follows is the endeavour of one hospital chaplain to enter into dialogue with a number of doctors and ethicists who are currently involved in the fields of human experimentation, organ transplantation, brain death, handicapped infants, and human fertilization and embryology — the additional problems of abortion and euthanasia are indirectly related to some of the latter concerns. It is to be hoped that it will serve as a useful resource for hospital chaplains, parish priests and ministers who wish to undertake further study of the problems outlined, and enable them to contribute constructively to on-going dialogue and debate.

Obviously in a study of this nature and scope it has been necessary to consult with many persons eminent in their respective fields. To them I extend my grateful thanks and their names are listed here:

Arnold Aldis, FRCS, MRCS, LRCP, Late Postgraduate Dean and Director, Postgraduate Medicine, University of Wales

Association for Spina Bifida and Hydrocephalus, Tavistock Square, London

The Very Revd Peter Baelz, MA, BD, DD, The Deanery, Durham

A. D. Barnes, ChM, MB, ChB, FRCS, Consultant Surgeon, Queen Elizabeth Hospital, Birmingham

R. W. Beard, MD, FRCOG, DObst, Professor of Obstetrics and

Gynaecology, Adviser, House of Commons Social Services Select Committee, St Mary's Hospital Medical School, London

A. Caroline Berry, PhD, Clinical Geneticist, Guy's Hospital Medical School, London

Michael Bewick, FRCS, Consultant Surgeon, Guy's Hospital, London

Sir Douglas Black, MD, PRCP, President, Royal College of Physicians, London. Formerly Professor of Medicine, University of Manchester

Martin Bobrow, DSc, MRCPath, Prince Philip Professor of Paediatric Research, Guy's Hospital Medical School

Colin Brewer, MRCS, LRCP, MRCPsych, DPM, Consultant Psychiatrist, Behavioural Science Unit, London

British Medical Association, Tavistock Square, London

R. P. Burden, MRCP, MRCS, LRCP, Consultant Physician, City Hospital, Nottingham

Roy Y. Calne, MA, MS, FRCS, FRS, Professor of Surgery, University of Cambridge

A. G. M. Campbell, FRCP, DCH, RCPS, Professor of Child Health, University of Aberdeen

Stuart Campbell, FRCOG, DObst., Professor of Obstetrics and Gynaecology, King's College Hospital Medical School, London

C. O. Carter, DM, FRCP, Professor of Clinical Genetics and Director, Clinical Genetics Unit, Institute of Child Health, London

P. A. F. Chalk, FRCS, FRCOG, Consultant Obstetrician and Gynaecologist, Royal Free Hospital, London

Iain Chalmers, MSc, MRCS, LRCP, MFCM, MRCOG, DCH, Director, National Perinatal Epidemiology Unit, Radcliffe Infirmary, Oxford

Christian Medical Fellowship, Waterloo Road, London

C. S. Clayden, MD, MRCS, LRCP, MRCP, Senior Lecturer in Paediatrics, St Thomas' Hospital Medical School, London

Ian Craft, FRCS, LRCP, MRCOG, Director, Gynaecology, Cromwell Hospital, London

Richard Cook, FRCS, Consultant Paediatric Surgeon, Royal Liverpool Children's Hospital & Alder Hey Children's Hospital, Liverpool

G. Crompton, MRCP, FFCM, DPH, DObst, RCOG, Chief Medical Officer, Welsh Office, Cardiff

Michael Denham, MD, FRCP, MRCS, LRCP, DCH, DObst, RCOG, Consultant Geriatrician, Northwick Park Hospital and Clinical Research Centre, Harrow

Eugene Diamond, MD, Professor of Pediatrics, Loyola University Stritch School of Medicine, Chicago, USA

H.M. Dick, MD, FRCP, MRCPath, Consultant in Clinical Immunology, Royal Infirmary, Glasgow

Brian Donald, BA, PhD, FHA, Council for Professions Supplementary to Medicine, Park House, London

Down's Children's Association, Quinborne Centre, Birmingham

Raymond S. Duff, MD, Associate Professor of Pediatrics, Yale University School of Medicine, Connecticut, USA

The Revd Canon G. R. Dunstan, MA, Hon DD, FSA, Department of Theology, University of Exeter

H. B. Eckstein, MD, MChir, FRCS, Consultant Paediatric Surgeon, Queen Mary's Hospital, Carshalton, and Hospital for Sick Children, Great Ormond Street, London

R. G. Edwards, PhD, DSc, Physiological Laboratory, University of Cambridge, Bourn Hall, Cambridge

Peter C. Elwood, MD, FRCP, FFCM, DPH, Director, MRC Epidemiology Research Unit (South Wales), Cardiff

Alan E. H. Emery, MD, PhD, DSc, FRCP, MFCM, FRS, Professor of Human Genetics, University of Edinburgh

T. A. H. English, MA, LRCP, FRCS, Consultant Cardiothoracic Surgeon, Papworth and Addenbrooke's Hospital, Cambridge

Ralph C. Evans, FRCP, DCH, Consultant Paediatrician, University Hospital of Wales, Cardiff

D. Wainwright Evans, MA, MD, FRCP, DCH, Consultant Cardiologist, East Anglian Regional Health Authority

Oswald Fernando, FRCS, Consultant Surgeon, Department of Nephrology and Transplantation, Royal Free Hospital, London

Joseph Fletcher, Visiting Professor of Biomedical Ethics, School of Medicine, University of Virginia, USA

R. F. R. Gardner, FRCOG, DObst, Consultant Obstetrician and Gynaecologist, Sunderland Health Authority

John Garfield, FRCP, FRCS, Consultant Neurosurgeon, Wessex Regional Health Authority

Charles F. George, MD, FRCP, Professor of Clinical Pharmacology, University of Southampton

Jonathan Glover, MA, BPhil, Fellow and Tutor in Philosophy, New College, Oxford

Janet Goodall, FRCP, MRCS, DObst, RCOG, DCH, Consultant Paediatrician, City General Hospital, Stoke-on-Trent

Peter Gray, FRCP, DCH, Professor of Child Health, Welsh National School of Medicine, Cardiff

G. A. Gresham, MA, MD, FRCPath, Professor of Morbid Anatomy and Histology, University of Cambridge

John Guillebaud, FRCS, MRCOG, Senior Lecturer Academic Unit, Middlesex Hospital, London

The Most Revd John Habgood, MA, PhD, DD, Archbishop of York

Peter Harper, MA, DM, FRCP, Professor of Medical Genetics, Welsh National School of Medicine, Cardiff

Rodney Harris, FRCP, FRCPath, Professor of Medical Genetics and Director, Department of Medical Genetics, University of Manchester

Heart-Transplant Patient

Bryan Hibbard, PhD, MD, MRCS, FRCOG, DObst, Professor of Obstetrics and Gynaecology, Welsh National School of Medicine

John Hinton, MD, DPM, FRCP, FRCPsych, Professor of Psychiatry, Middlesex Hospital Medical School, London

Fr Gerard J. Hughes, SJ, Heythrop College, University of London

Human Rights Society, Walpole Street, London

Jack Insley, FRCP, DCH, Consultant Paediatrician, Infant Development Unit, Queen Elizabeth Medical Centre, Birmingham

Bryan Jennett, MD, FRCS, Professor of Neurosurgery, Institute of Neurological Sciences, Southern General Hospital, Glasgow

Hugh Jolly, MA, FRCP, MRCS, DCH: Late Consultant Paediatrician, Department of Paediatrics, Charing Cross Hospital, London

Ian Kennedy, LLM, Professor of Medical Law and Ethics, University of London

C. Everett Koop, MD, Surgeon General of the Public Health Service, Washington DC, USA

Keith E. Kirkham, MA, PhD, Assistant Director (Administration), Clinical Research Centre, Harrow

Desmond Laurence, MD, FRCP, Professor of Pharmacology and Therapeutics, University College School of Medicine, London

Michael Laurence, DSc, FRCP, FRCPath, Professor of Paediatric Research, Head of Regional Cytogenetics Service, Wales, Welsh National School of Medicine, Cardiff

B.A. Lieberman, MRCOG, Consultant Gynaecologist and Obstetrician, St. Mary's Hospital, Manchester

LIFE, Leamington Spa, Warwickshire

Linacre Centre, London

Gillian Lockwood, Clinical Medical Student, John Radcliffe Hospital, Oxford

Michael Lockwood, MA, DPhil, Staff Tutor in Philosophy, Department for External Studies, University of Oxford

John Lorber, MD, FRCP, Professor (Emeritus) and Head of Department, Department of Paediatrics, Sheffield

L. C. Lum, FRACP, Late Physician, Papworth Hospital, Cambridge

Bruce MacGillivray, FRCP, Dean, Royal Free Hospital School of Medicine, London

Robert Mahler, FRCP, Consultant Physician, Northwick Park Hospital and MRC Clinical Research Centre, Harrow

Fr John Mahoney, SJ, Heythrop College, University of London

N. P. Mallick, FRCP, Physician i/c Department of Renal Medicine, Manchester Royal Infirmary

J. K. Mason, CBE, MD, FRCPath, DMJ, Professor of Forensic Medicine, University of Edinburgh

Thomas Mawdsley, MA, DObst, RCOG, Clinical Assistant, Alder Hey Children's Hospital, Liverpool

Mary G. McGeown, PhD, MD, FRCP, Consultant Medical Urologist and Physician in Admin Charge, Renal Unit, Belfast City and Royal Victoria Hospitals, Belfast

L. Mettler (and members of Group), Professor, Klinikum Der Christian-Albrechts-Universitat, Kiel, W. Germany

George Mitchell, MB, ChB, Senior Lecturer, Department of Pharmacology, Welsh National School of Medicine, Cardiff

G. D. Mitchell, Professor, Institute of Population Studies, University of Exeter

The Revd E. Garth Moore, Fellow of Corpus Christi College, Cambridge; of Gray's Inn, Barrister-at-Law; Chairman of the Legal Advisory Commission of the Church of England

Peter Morris, MA, PhD, FACS, FRCS, Nuffield Professor of Surgery, University of Oxford

Lars Nilsson (and members of Group), Department of Obstetrics & Gynaecology, University of Goteberg, Sweden

The Revd Canon Oliver O'Donovan, MA, PhD, Regius Professor of Moral and Pastoral Theology, Christ Church, Oxford

Christopher Pallis, DM, FRCP, Reader (Emeritus) in Neurology, Royal Postgraduate Medical School, University of London

Victor Parsons, DM, FRCP, Physician i/c Renal Dialysis Unit, Dulwich Hospital, London

Sir John Peel, KCVO, FRCP, FRCS, FRCOG, Past President, Royal College of Obstetricians and Gynaecologists

Pope John XXIII Center, Missouri, USA

Prospect, Warlingham, Surrey

Jean Purdy, Bourn Hall, Cambridge

Paul Ramsey, Harrington Spear Paine Professor of Religion, Princeton University, New Jersey, USA

M.A.C. Ridler, PhD, MIBiol, Consultant Cytogeneticist, Kennedy-Galton Centre for Clinical Genetics, Harperbury Hospital, Shenley, Herts

Alan Richens, PhD, FRCP, Professor of Pharmacology and Therapeutics, Welsh National School of Medicine, Cardiff

Sir Gordon Robson, CBE, FRCS, FFARCS, Professor of Anaesthetics, Royal Postgraduate Medical School, University of London

John Scanlon, MD, Director of Neonatology, Columbia Hospital for Women, Washington DC, USA

M. Seabright, PhD, MRCPath, FIBiol, (and members of Group), Head of Unit, Wessex Regional Cytogenetics Unit, General Hospital, Salisbury

James Seakins, MA, PhD, Senior Lecturer in Clinical Chemistry, Institute of Child Health, London

R. A. Sells, MA, FRCS, LRCP, Consultant Surgeon & Director, Renal Transplant Unit, Royal Liverpool Hospital; Clinical Lecturer, University of Liverpool

Anthony Shaw, MD, Director, Department of Pediatric Surgery; Clinical Professor of Surgery, University of California School of Medicine, USA

William A. Silverman, MD, Late Professor of Clinical Pediatrics, Columbia University. Director, The Premature Nursery Babies Hospital, New York, USA

Peter Singer, Professor of Philosophy and Director of the Centre for Human Bioethics. Chairman, Department of Philosophy, Monash University, Melbourne, Australia

Maurice Slapak, MChir, FRCS, FACS, Co-Director, Wessex Regional Transplant Unit, St Mary's Hospital, Portsmouth

Eliot Slater (RIP 1983), MA, MD, FRCP, MRCS, FRCPsych, DPM, Late Director, MRC Psychiatric Genetics Unit, National Hospital, London

Robert Snowden, PhD, Institute of Population Studies, University of Exeter

E. Southern, MRC Mammalian Genome Unit, Edinburgh

Society for the Protection of the Unborn Child, London

Alec I. Speiers, Royal Women's Hospital, Victoria, Australia

Sir John Stallworthy, FRCS, FRCOG, Emeritus Nuffield Professor of Obstetrics and Gynaecology, University of Oxford

Carson Strong, Assistant Professor and Director, Human Values and Ethics, Memphis, Tennessee, USA

M. Super, MD, MSc, FRCP, DCH, RCPS, Consultant Clinical Geneticist and Hon. Lecturer, Salford Health Authority

Valerie Thompson, FRCOG, FRCS, LRCP, Consultant Gynaecologist, Royal Free Hospital, London

Bernard Towers, MB, ChB, Professor of Pediatrics and Anatomy, University of California, Los Angeles, USA

Robert Twycross, DM, FRCP, Consultant Physician, Sir Michael Sobell House, The Churchill Hospital, Headington, Oxford

Duncan Vere, FRCP, Professor of Therapeutics, University of London

Voluntary Euthanasia Society, Kensington, London

Owen L. Wade, CBE, FRCP, FRCPI, Dean of the Faculty of

Medicine and Dentistry; Professor of Therapeutics and Clinical Pharmacology, University of Birmingham

William Walters, MBBS, PhD, FRCOG, FRACOG, Assistant Professor, Department of Obstetricians and Gynaecologists, Monash University, Melbourne, Australia

The Revd Keith Ward, MA, BLitt, Professor of Moral and Social Theology, King's College, London

William B. Weil Jr, MD, Professor of Pediatrics, Michigan State University, Michigan, USA

Margaret White, DObst, RCOG, Late Assistant MOH, Borough of Croydon

A. W. Wilkinson, ChM, FRCSE, Professor (Emeritus) of Paediatric Surgery, Institute of Child Health, University of London

R. Williamson, MSc, PhD, Professor of Biochemistry, St Mary's Hospital Medical School, London

P. J. E. Wilson, FRCS, Consultant Neurosurgeon, Department of Surgical Neurology, Morriston Hospital, Swansea

Sir Gordon Wolstenholme, CBE, LLD, MD, FRCP, MRCS, Late Master Society of Apothecaries, London; Director, Ciba Foundation

World Council of Churches, Geneva, Switzerland

1
Human Experimentation

Human experimentation is as old as medicine itself; it is the modern methods and techniques of carrying out such experiments that are comparatively new. If the physician is denied the right to experiment he might as well give up his medicine, for medical progress can only be made by means of experimentation. It is essential for both scientific progress and the welfare of mankind. If Jenner had not been prepared to give the boy, James Phipps, cowpox and then subsequently attempt to give him smallpox, the science of immunology would not have reached its state today. If William Withering had not tried out the effects of foxglove infusion on his dropsical patients, countless thousands of sufferers from heart disease would not have had the benefit of digitalis.[1] Many such benefits have been dominantly the result of human experimentation. Indeed in some instances it may be considered unethical not to experiment; for example, to retest traditional treatments that may have been accepted in the past. The modern teaching hospital is geared towards the dual orientation of treatment and research, and the physician of today places greater and greater emphasis on scientific investigations. Addressing medical editors in Rome in September 1954, Pope Pius XII recognized that medicine could not do without human experimentation: 'Que la recherche et la pratique médicale ne puissent se passer de toute experiméntation sur l'homme vivant, on le comprend sans peine.'

Medicine today benefits greatly from the experiments of the past, and today's experiment becomes tomorrow's commonplace.

In one sense even ordinary routine treatment is experimental, for each individual patient is a unique being, personally and physiologically. Reactions of patients will differ and it is often extremely difficult to draw the line between 'treatment' and 'trial', or to state or explain when experimentation ceases. The Declaration of Helsinki (vide p. 207) helps to distinguish between trial and treatment by following the principles that 'the doctor can combine medical research with professional care, the objective being the acquisition of new medical knowledge, only to the extent that medical research is justifiable by its potential diagnostic or therapeutic value for the patient'. Strictly speaking every therapeutic procedure may be considered a fresh experiment, for as Sir Geoffrey Jefferson once put it: 'The prescription of even rest in bed for two or three weeks, or of a bottle of cough mixture, are experiments, the results of which deserve closer observations and quantitative analyses than they get'.[2]

What then, I asked a number of physicians, are the characteristics that differentiate human experimentation from ordinary therapeutic or surgical intervention, and who is to decide when standard practice becomes experimentation? Professor Charles George explained:

> 'The main difference is that greater emphasis is placed upon objective measurement to assess the progress of the illness and its response to treatment. In addition, there may be a comparison made with an inert placebo treatment. Although in theory such patients would be at a disadvantage, in practice they tend to enjoy a better standard of care because of the greater interest shown and the time devoted to them. Standard practice can rarely, if ever, be regarded as experimentation. By contrast, experimentation tends to become tomorrow's standard practice.'

Professor Duncan Vere outlined some of the characteristics of an experiment:

> '1. Certain applied constraints which lie outside ordinary practice:
>   (a) changes in the order, timing, and nature of treatments.
>   (b) enrolment of matched controls.
>   (c) involvement of comparable groups rather than individuals.
> 2. A primary aim to increase knowledge rather than simply to benefit the individual.'

On the question as to who is to decide when standard practice becomes experimentation Professor Duncan Vere gave as his opinion that

> 'as the transition from experience to experiment is well understood in general by medical staff, it seems reasonable to leave the decision to them.'

An interesting viewpoint from the American scene was given by Dr William B. Weil:

> 'The decision is probably made by the physician or the agency of government (FDA), or often third party insurers in this country — i.e. will it be paid for?'

Human experimentation can be classified into three different categories:
(1) That designed to benefit the patient himself; (2) that which attempts to explore physiological or clinical problems about disease processes which may only remotely benefit the patient concerned, but may benefit others in the future; and (3) that concerned with volunteers with no personal individual benefit but of potential value for the advancement of medicine.

The subject of human experimentation is both highly complex and open to a great deal of misunderstanding. To the non-medical it has connotations of either the factual atrocities of Nazi concentration camps in World War Two, or the fictional and horror film images of Frankenstein or Jekyll and Hyde. As one physician put it to me: 'The phrase "human experimentation" conjures up an image of demented doctors working in a chamber of horrors!' In the minds of some it spells out malpractice, and the mass media are inclined to refer emotively to 'human guinea-pigs!'

As I discussed these concerns with Professor Owen Wade, he had some very important comments to make:

> 'I think one of the underlying problems which effects all our thinking about experimental work is related to professionalism. What is a professional man? What are the responsibilities of a professional man? How does a professional man behave? In a sense, the community, the

public, or the person who is sick, is best protected if we have a medical profession which consists of people with high professional standards. This is a much greater protection to the community than laws, regulations or guidelines, because once you have a law or regulation then it is always possible for people to get around legislation or get around the law. No legal system can substitute for the high quality of personal behaviour by the individual physician or surgeon, whoever he may be. So I think the most important protection is the calibre of people we have as doctors.'

He went on to make some encouraging remarks:

'I feel it is of tremendous help to those of us who work in hospitals or those of us who are physicians and surgeons to have people like you, hospital chaplains, who are outside our profession yet nevertheless observe us fairly closely and who can speak for us. Obviously if we speak for ourselves we are somewhat suspect. One of the problems at the moment seems to me to be that there is a strong reaction against the establishment. There are people who turn rather rudely away from what they term "conventional medicine". Very often in the criticisms that are made of medicine is the idea that doctors do not care. I feel very strongly about this. As a Dean of a Medical School I have 160 young students coming in every year. I am always very impressed just how concerned medical students and young doctors are about their patients. The dedication of the staff is enormous — not just doctors but nursing and other staff as well.'

International Declarations

As a result of the atrocities carried out in Nazi concentration camps in World War Two and revealed at the Nuremberg Trials, the Tribunal drew up on 19 August 1947, the first international declaration on research involving human subjects. Known as the Nuremberg Code, it sets out a ten-point declaration to serve as a guide to those carrying out research. It lays particular stress on the 'voluntary consent' (usually now referred to as 'informed consent') of the subject which it states as 'absolutely essential'.

The Helsinki Code with its recommendations guiding medical doctors in biomedical research involving human beings was adopted by the 18th World Medical Assembly (WMA), Helsinki, Finland, in 1964. It was later revised by the 29th World Medical Assembly, Tokyo, Japan, in 1975. It has been extended most recently in September, 1981, (*World Health Council for International Organizations of Medical Sciences. Proposed International Guidelines for Biomedical Research involving Human Subjects*, Geneva, WSO 1982). The Code has three main sections devoted to (1) basic principles, (2) medical research combined with professional care (clinical research), and (3) non-therapeutic biomedical research involving human subjects (non-clinical biomedical research).

In the 1975 revision of the Code its scope was broadened from 'clinical research' to 'biomedical research.' Important new provisions in the extended code of 1981 were that experimental protocols for research with human subjects 'should be transmitted to a specially appointed independent Committee for consideration, comment and guidance'. (1.2); that such protocols 'should always contain a statement of the ethical considerations involved and should indicate that the principles enunciated in the present Declaration are complied with' (1.12), and that reports on 'experimentation not in accordance with the principles laid down in this Declaration should not be accepted for publication' (1.8). The revised Declaration (known as Helsinki II) now supersedes both the Nuremberg Code and the original Declaration of Helsinki (Helsinki I, 1964). The main formulae of the Codes or Declarations state that no research can be performed on human subjects without voluntary informed consent, and that experiments are to be carried out only with the expectation of fruitful results for the good of society, and of benefits that should outweigh any potential risks.

The Medical Research Council (MRC) published its statement, *Responsibility in Investigations on Human Subjects* in 1962–63. It makes a very important distinction 'between procedures undertaken as part of patient care which are intended to contribute to the benefit of the individual patient, by treat-

ment, prevention or assessment, and those procedures which
are undertaken either on patients or on healthy subjects solely
for the purpose of contributing to medical knowledge and are
not themselves designed to benefit the particular individual on
whom they are performed'.[3]

Although the various codes offer authoritative guidelines
they actually differ in their advice concerning clinical research
which is not designed to be of direct benefit to the subject
(non-therapeutic research: NTR). It should be emphasized
that these codes or guidelines do not have the force of law. No
matter how significant or important these Codes or Declarations may be they can never be a substitute for the basic trust
and confidence between doctor and patient.

Informed Consent

Basic to the whole subject of human experimentation is consent, designed to uphold the ethical principle of respect for
persons, and the sanctity of human life; to accord the patient
the status of a human being, as an end, not a means. A person
has the right to decide what is to be done to his body. For
example, a surgeon who operates on a patient without his or
her consent commits an assault for which he is liable to
damages. (There would, of course, be obvious exceptions in
the case of accidents or emergencies.) The patient must be
allowed to make decisions and to exercise choice on matters
which affect him. The principle of 'informed consent' recognizes the patient's dignity and integrity. Its aim is to achieve a
partnership between individuals (investigator and subject) of
common understanding and intentions. Paul Ramsey, the
Protestant theologian and ethicist, describes (1971) 'informed
consent' as representing 'a convenantal bond between
consenting man and consenting man (that) makes them . . .
joint adventurers in medical care and progress'.[4]

The Helsinki Declaration plainly affirms that 'clinical
research on a human being cannot be undertaken without his
free consent after he has been fully informed; if he is legally
incompetent, the consent of the legal guardian should be
procured'. It states that the interests of the individual must
take priority over those of society. 'Concern for the interests of
the subject must always prevail over the interests of science

and society' (1.5). 'In research on man, the interest of science and society should never take precedence over considerations related to the well-being of the subject' (111.4).

To be valid consent must be free of coercion, and the subject aware of the dangers and alternatives as well as of the benefits of the experiment. Absolute importance must be given to such willing consent. The patient should understand fully what is to be done, why it is to be done, and the discomfort and risk entailed. 'Informed consent' can become a complicated and complex problem, for the patient must be partner as well as participant. There is often the difficulty of communicating medical information to a layman. As far as is possible the subject has truly to understand the purpose, the discomforts, the risks, however remote, and the benefits of the work at hand. Full and informed consent is mandatory to human experimentation as far as this can be achieved. Indeed such full and informed consent is not only an ethical but also a legal requirement.

The investigator must be prepared to answer any queries raised by the subject and also ready to disclose alternative drugs or procedures which are available, whilst the patient must be a partner in the decisions of determining what shall be done to him and also the final determinant of whether he participates and under what conditions. As one doctor described it: 'A subject must be neither "blinded by science" nor "pressured", but given a "fair go!".'

The conditions of the procedure, the risks and benefits are to be clearly outlined in a language and terms the patient can fully understand, for 'informed consent' must exist throughout the conduct of the study, not simply at its commencement. The Nuremberg Code makes this plain: 'The nature, duration and purpose of the experiment, the method and means by which it is conducted, all inconveniences and hazards reasonably to be expected, and the effects upon his health or person which may possibly come from his participation in the experiment.' This is to help him make the most 'understanding and enlightened decision.'

Yet how 'informed' can or should 'informed consent' be? Ingelfinger (1972) states that 'it would be impractical and probably unethical for the investigator to present the nearly endless list of all possible contingencies; in fact he may not himself be aware of every untoward thing that might happen. Excessive detail, moreover, usually enhances the subject's confusion. . . . Incapacitated and hospitalized because of illness, frightened by strange and impersonal routines, and fearful for his health and perhaps life, he is far from exercising a free power of choice when the person to whom he anchors all his hopes asks, "Say, you wouldn't mind, would you, if you joined some of the other patients . . . and helped us to carry out some very important research we are doing?"[5] The British Medical Association (BMA) in their *Handbook of Medical Ethics* (BMA, London, 1980, p. 25) outlines the situation thus: 'Most patients trust their doctors and will consent to any proposal. Experimental procedures are nearly always too technical for patients or non-experts to understand.'

Unconscious and subtle coercions on the part of the doctor/ investigator have closely to be watched (e.g. 'It would make a very good impression if I get this research paper done!'), and the emotional vulnerability of the patient (e.g. 'Anything for you, doctor!') has to be strictly protected. The only real protection the patient has is the conscience and compassion of the investigator, who should be highly competent and skilled. It goes without saying, too, that the experiment should be necessary and scientifically valid.

In the light of these issues I posed the question: How much information must patients be given? Can there ever be such a thing as 'fully informed' consent?

> 'Yes, there is fully informed consent,' stated Professor Duncan Vere, 'but it is seldom attained if the patient is not a medical or nursing or science graduate. However, *relevant* informed consent covers a much wider field; at least the aspects of risk and inconvenience which are relevant to the patient can be explained to any intelligent subject. Exceptions are the very young, the demented, the psychotic, the unconscious, and those for whom it may be damaging to disclose all relevant facts — for example, some instances of chemotherapy.'

According to John W. Scanlon:

> 'If one defines the patients' need to know in practical terms — reasonable risks, most serious complications,

etc. — then patients can be fully (not absolutely) informed.'

He went on to emphasize that

'this requires skill as an educator, honesty and candour about what is and is not known.'

There must often be risk, for if no risk is permissible then much research could not take place. The calculated risk must be weighed against the benefit gained. The evaluation of risk and benefit constitutes one of the major ethical dilemmas in human experimentation. It is generally agreed that only when the benefits outweigh the risks is such research ethical. The US Department of Health, Education and Welfare guidelines give the following definition: 'An individual is considered to be "at risk" if he may be exposed to the possibility of harm — physical, psychological, sociological, or other — as a consequence of any activity which goes beyond the application of those established and accepted methods necessary to meet his needs.'

Provided the subject knows and fully understands what his doctors are trying to do, is free to ask questions and seek advice, free to refuse or withdraw, then no real objection arises. What does cause some concern is whether the attempt at reasonable and adequate explanation to patients is always made. When the subject himself cannot give consent (infants, children, minors, mentally handicapped, relationship to physician) problems arise, but children or others can be represented by parents or legal guardians. The readiness of an investigator to experiment on himself is not necessarily a valid justification that an identical experiment is justifiable on a patient.

Difficulties over obtaining fully informed consent can sometimes arise in instances where the physician feels that the patient is not in a position to handle the emotional impact of being fully informed of the nature of his disease. For example, a patient suffering from a terminal illness, who has not been told of the diagnosis and its prognosis, is not able to give fully informed consent to experimental treatment unless told truthfully about his physical condition and its possible outcome. In such examples the physician may feel justified in withholding some information in order to avoid emotional distress, and to uphold the primary ethical demand — *'primum non nocere.'* In clinical experience it has been found that psychological states involving inability to cope with stress are associated with increased incidence and poorer prognosis of cancer.[6]

This withholding of fully adequate information, particularly about risks and dangers, is sometimes referred to as 'therapeutic privilege', and it is clear that requirements of informed consent cannot be absolute, and levels of non-disclosure are ethically and legally permissible. Is 'informed consent' then always necessary? A number of doctors were of the opinion that it was. Some wished to qualify their responses, while others gave a definite 'No'. Professor Duncan Vere pinpointed some situations where consent is not necessary:

> 'Where it is damaging to elicit it — for example some cases of cancer chemotherapy; where it cannot be elicited without altering the disease under study — some psychiatric trials (for example, in anxiety), and in trivial disorders and where treatment carried no risk.'

In no way, however, must this therapeutic privilege of non-disclosure be permitted to become an instrument of exploitation. The current editor of the *Journal of Medical Ethics*, Dr Raanan Gillon, outlines this admirably: 'the critical moral issue here seems to be whether or not patients may be deliberately deceived or lied to about their medical condition in order to save them distress. If this is an acceptable aspect of medical ethics (and it is certainly a maxim of many doctors' actions) then presumably it should be acceptable for research ethics committees to sanction it, and the Declaration of Helsinki should be amended accordingly. On the other hand an opposing view, also common within the medical profession, is that doctors must *not* lie to or deliberately deceive their patients, even though they should be sensitive about not thrusting *unwanted* truths at patients who, having been given genuine opportunities to ask about their condition, make it clear that they "don't want to know". The moral obligation not to lie or deliberately deceive is a general moral norm and is linked with the moral obligation to respect other people as autonomous agents — a respect which also leads to the view that people have a right to obtain medical information they desire about themselves, even if obtaining it will lead to distress.'[7]

From a point of personal interest I asked how far is it necessary for 'consent' to be a written document? Possibly it might provide a form of protection for both the 'subject' and the 'investigator'. Professor Owen Wade told me about his own practice:

> 'If I am going to get informed consent, I much prefer to call in a sister or staff-nurse and say, "I'm going to speak to Mr X here. I want to explain to him what we are going to do, or what we want to try out, and I want you to listen. If he agrees I want to be quite sure that, when he does agree, he has understood what I have said. You will be a much better judge of whether he is understanding than I am". What I personally prefer is that I have a statement which is signed by the sister/staff-nurse saying, "Professor Wade explained the protocol of this or that experiment to Mr X, who agreed to take part in this and in my opinion understood to what he was agreeing". I know from a lawyer's point of view it probably covers me much better if I were to say to the patient: "Here's a form. I want you to sign it because we are going to do some tests on you. Will you sign it?" Then the patient signs it usually very readily, but I much prefer the other method. From my point of view as a professional man, I feel I am getting a much better acquiescence from the patient by that method, but I think you will find the practice and procedure varies.'

Professor Charles George confirmed the views of Professor Wade:

> 'Written consent is becoming a matter of tradition rather than contributing anything in terms of legal protection. All it means is that the patient signed the piece of paper! Unless the procedure is explained by the investigator in the presence of an independent witness, I doubt if written consent has any more value than verbal consent. Written information sheets are, however, one way of

allowing the patient to think further about what is involved and to generate questions before he/she finally participates (or declines).'

Experiments on Children

The subject of experimentation on children evokes strong emotions and public reaction is often ambivalent. While the participation of children is indispensable for research on diseases of childhood and conditions to which children are particularly susceptible (e.g. the work that has brought about the virtual elimination of some of the infectious diseases — diphtheria, polio and measles, etc.), it is axiomatic that they should never be subjects of research that might equally well be carried out on adults. As Professor Alan Richens put it to me:

> 'If you banned experimentation in children then you wouldn't have many advances because the only way you are going to make advances is to use the people who are going to use the drugs. Children handle drugs in a very different manner from adults; their metabolic rate is faster; they break down drugs much more quickly. They may produce different metabolites and the only way we've got information about this is by doing experimental work on children. Had we not done that we would still be in the dark ages with therapeutics in children.'

Ethical and legal implications which cause controversy concern the obtaining of consent for non-therapeutic experimentation on infants and children, for such a vulnerable group must clearly be protected from exploitation as research subjects. The 'golden rule' in its positive form, 'do unto others as you would have them do unto you', still has some relevance as A. G. M. Campbell (1974) indicates: 'Though this can be a fallible guide, the investigator should ask himself as honestly as he can if this is an experiment to which he would freely submit his own child if appropriate. Are the risks that small? If he feels hesitant or uncomfortable about this question he should not proceed. His patients have a right to expect that sort of protection.'[8] Children have to rely on the protection of their parents who carry a heavy burden of responsibility when decisions have to be made.

A 1975 Circular of the Department of Health and Social Security drew attention to 'the Royal College of Physicians' recommendation that clinical research investigations of children or mentally handicapped adults which is not of direct benefit to the patient may be conducted only when the procedures entail negligible risk or discomfort, subject to the provisions of any common and statute law prevailing at the time and with the consent of the parent or guardian.' The following is an extract from the Report of the Medical Research Council for 1962–63 which emphasizes the practical difficulties in the interpretation of ethical standards and codes, which serve only as guides and do not relieve members of the medical profession from criminal and civil responsibilities under the law of the land:

'The situation in respect of minors and mentally subnormal or mentally disordered persons is of particular difficulty. In the strict view of the law, parents and guardians of minors cannot give consent on their behalf to any procedures which are of no particular benefit to them and which may carry some risk of harm. Whilst English law does not fix any arbitary age in this context, it may safely be assumed that the Courts will not regard a child of 12 years or under (or 14 years or under for boys in Scotland) as having the capacity to consent to any procedure which may involve him in an injury . . . In the case of those who are mentally subnormal or mentally disordered the reality of the consent given will fall to be judged by similar criteria to those which apply to the making of a will, contracting a marriage or otherwise taking decisions which have legal force as well as moral and social implications. When true consent in this sense cannot be obtained, procedures which are of no direct benefit and which might carry a risk of harm to the subject should not be undertaken.

Even when true consent has been given by a minor or mentally subnormal or mentally disordered person, consideration of ethics and prudence still require that, if possible, the assent of parents or guardians or relatives, as the case may be, should be obtained.'

An important distinction has to be made between therapeutic research which is undertaken for the direct benefit of the subject and where the possible benefits are considered to outweigh the risks, and non-therapeutic experimentation where the benefits, if any, would occur to others and the subject personally is offered no immediate benefit (see above). Non-therapeutic research is defined as of no benefit to the subject but may benefit the health and welfare of other children or adults, and may add to basic biological knowledge.

The consent of parents, proxy consent, is morally valid only if it can be presumed that if the child could consent for himself, he would do so since such therapy is considered for his benefit. The legality of such consent has been questioned. The Department of Health and Social Security (DHSS) states that 'the position in law is that no parent or guardian of a child of tender years is entitled to give consent to any procedure which is not for the benefit of the child.'[9] This view was challenged by P. D. G. Skegg, Faculty of Law, University of Oxford, who advocated (1977) that harmless investigations with the consent of the ethical committee, the paediatrician in charge, and, above all, the mother, are, in his view, legal.[10] Professor Gerald Dworkin (1978) supports Skegg and submits that it is probably perfectly legal for a parent to consent to a procedure on a child which is not of direct benefit to him, provided the study is approved by an ethical committee and there is no, or minimal, risk to the child.[11]

Another element which has to be carefully considered is that of risk, which is always a factor, no matter how slight, in all medical research. The risk benefit ratio attempts to contrast the degree of benefit resulting from a research in relation to the risks of discomfort or pain to the participant. Questions arise about the protection and rights of a child and the authority of the parents.

In 1978 the British Paediatric Association set up a working party on Ethics of Research on Children, and issued guidelines to ethical committees considering research involving children. Among the premises accepted by the working party are that research involving children is important for the benefit of all children and should be supported and encouraged and conducted in an ethical manner; that research should never be done on children if the same investigation could be done on adults, and that research which involves a child and is of no benefit to that child (non-therapeutic research) is not necessarily either unethical or illegal (both Skegg and Dworking are mentioned in support of NTR on children).[12]

The moral problems primarily concern non-therapeutic research, where there is no benefit to the person concerned to offset possible risk. A number of theologians (e.g. Fletcher, McCormick) consider that consent implied, presumed or proxy, is valid for clinical research where the risk is so minimal and remote that a normal and informed individual would be presupposed to give ready consent.[13] On the other hand, Paul Ramsey adopts a much firmer line and denies the validity of proxy consent in non-beneficial experiments on children. Ramsey (1970) argues: 'To attempt to consent for a child to be made an experimental subject is to treat a child as not a child. It is to treat him as if he were an adult person who has consented to become a joint adventurer in the common cause of medical research. If the grounds for this are alleged to be the presumptive or implied consent of the child, that must simply be characterized as a violent and a false presumption', and he concludes simply that 'no parent is morally competent to consent that his child shall be subjected to hazardous or other experiments having no diagnostic or therapeutic significance for the child himself'.[14]

When I discussed the problem with Professor Ian Kennedy at King's College, London, he confessed how difficult and delicate a subject it was:

> 'Probably the law, (and I mean my view of what it is), now seems to be not so much that parents must always act in the best interests of the child, but that they may not act against the interests of the child, and that is quite different. In other words, they must not act against the interests of the child, but their actions need not necessarily be in the *best* interests of the child. I speak generally now of therapeutic and non-therapeutic experimentation. If you apply this test to non-therapeutic research you can see that there might be circumstances in which a parent might volunteer a child because there might be

peripheral social benefits to the child. In my view a
parent in law is not debarred from volunteering his child
for certain things, but may only volunteer his child when
the risk to that child is of a minimal nature, for example,
a pinprick or a prick in the ear to take blood. The better
approach is to classify risks rather than have a blanket
prohibition. Indeed, a lot of the problems of non-
therapeutic research are due to establishing normal
levels. You can't do research until you find out what the
norm is, so you need normal children. And where the risk
to the child is minimal, I would suggest that parents may
properly volunteer their children for such research.'

I asked Ian Kennedy, if parents can give consent for therapeutic research, why should there be limits as regards non-
therapeutic research?

'Because the key is in the word "therapeutic",' he
replied. 'The key is in the notion that although it be
research — research meaning a part of a project which is
scientifically valid and which will produce generalizable
knowledge — it is also therapeutic; namely, it is intended
to treat this particular individual and will only be
employed when other or better treatment is not available
which would solve the problem. It will, therefore, inevit-
ably or prima facie at least, be in the best interests of the
child for the parent to volunteer. Indeed it would be
arguable whether the parent could refuse. On the other
hand, non-therapeutic research refers to interventions
which are not intended as treatment. Indeed the child
may be healthy. I think that, even where the research is
non-therapeutic, the parent can volunteer the child for
minimal risks because, as against the benefit which may
be gained, the risks are not very great. I used to hold the
view that parents couldn't volunteer the child even in
such circumstances, but now I am persuaded that if you
can categorize the risks adequately, and it involves fairly
sophisticated psychological assessment, I am happy to
go along with the view the Americans take — that a
parent may consent to research on his child when the
research involves only minimal risks.'

The use of children who are incompetent to consent in non-therapeutic research is indeed an extremely difficult and complex ethical problem. Such experimental protocol must be subjected to careful ethical committee scrutiny, with the assurance that the knowledge to be gained by the experiment can be obtained only by experimentation involving children; that it involves the minimal or no risk or discomfort to the child; that the experiment would provide significant and essential new knowledge, and, of course, have parental consent which is mandatory from parents who are aware of what is contemplated, understand the nature of the experiment and have had a genuine opportunity to object.

Research on Fetuses and Fetal Material
The most important ethical problems regarding research on fetuses and/or fetal material revolve around a number of issues: the rights of a mother, a fetus which is going to be aborted, or a fetus which is presumed defective, and the personality of the fetus. There appears to be a great variety of viewpoints in all these matters, from a firm and definite 'No' in circumstances where the fetus would be exposed to any risk or 'offensive touching', to the extreme point of view in which it would be considered unethical not to carry out research on unwanted fetuses for the benefit of those which are wanted.

Normally fetal experimentation is seen to be justifiable only where the abortion is spontaneous, or is considered to be morally legitimate. It is indispensable for some medical research to use human fetal tissue or indeed the whole fetus itself, but where such research is undertaken it should only be on fetuses that would, by common consent, have no hope at all of continued extra–uterine existence. (John Enders and Thomas Weller were awarded the Nobel Prize in 1965 for their work in growing poliomyolitis virus in cells cultured from human fetal tissues.) It goes without saying that in no circumstances should potentially viable fetuses be used for experimentation.

It was as a result of a speech to Parliament by Mr Norman St John-Stevas, MP, giving prominence to reports of the commercial sale of human fetuses for research purposes in Great Britain that an advisory group was appointed to draw up regulations, chaired by Sir John Peel of The Royal College of Obstetrics and Gynaecology. The Report entitled *The Use of Fetuses and Fetal Material for Research* was issued in May 1972 (HMSO Department of Health and Social Security Scottish Home and Health Department Welsh Office). The recommended Code of Practice includes the following:

1. Where the fetus is viable after separation from the mother it is unethical to carry out any experiments on it which are inconsistent with treatment necessary to promote its life.
2. The minimal limit of viability for human fetuses should be regarded as 20 weeks gestational age. This corresponds to a weight of approximately 400–500 grammes.
3. The use of the whole dead fetus or tissues from dead fetuses for medical research is permissible subject to the following conditions:
   (a) The provisions of the Human Tissue Act (see p. 210) are observed where applicable;
   (b) Where the provisions of the Human Tissue Act do not apply there is no known objection on the part of the parent who has had an opportunity to declare any wishes about the disposal of the fetus;
   (c) Dissection of the dead fetus or experiments on the fetus or fetal material do not occur in the operating theatre or place of delivery;
   (d) There is no monetary exchange for fetuses or fetal material;
   (e) Full records are kept by the relevant institution.
4. The use of the whole pre-viable fetus is permissible provided that:
   (a) The conditions in paragraph 3 above are observed;
   (b) Only fetuses weighing less than 300 grammes are used;
   (c) The responsibility for deciding that the fetus is in a category which may be used for this type of research rests with the medical attendants at its

birth and never with the intending research worker;

(d) Such research is only carried out in departments directly related to a hospital and with the direct sanction of its ethical committee;

(e) Before permitting such research the ethical committee satisfies itself:

(i) on the validity of the research; (ii) that the required information cannot be obtained in any other way; and (iii) that the investigators have the necessary facilities and skill.

5. It is unethical to administer drugs or carry out any procedures during pregnancy with the deliberate intent of ascertaining the harm that they might do to the fetus.

It is important to distinguish between the viable and the non-viable fetus and the distinction which must be made, in considering research in dead fetal matter, between the still-born child and the fetus. A child is still-born if it is produced after the twenty-eighth week and if it has not breathed or shown signs of life. The fetus which is stillborn may be legally used for scientific purposes.

Clinical Trials

The most common form of experimentation on human subjects is the administration of new drugs. It is estimated that approximately five hundred drugs enter the market each year, and every time a doctor administers a drug he can be said to be experimenting for he cannot be aware of all the potentialities for good or ill. (It should be explained that many of the new products are formulations of existing drugs and do not require elaborate tests in human beings.) The requirement to test all *new* medicinal substances, in the first instance in laboratory animals, and ultimately in human beings, is enacted in the Medicines Act (1968). The World Health Organization, in its *International Guidelines for Biomedical Research on Human Beings* (Geneva, 1982), also recognizes the need to assess the safety of medicines intended for use in man. It lays down its own requirements and codes for biomedical research in man and that such research 'must conform to generally accepted scientific principles'. It should be based on adequately performed animal experiments and thorough knowledge of the scientific literature.[15]

Clinical trials are defined as scientific studies by which the benefit of one or more medical treatments are assessed. These may be drugs and vaccines, surgical operations or physical treatments such as physiotherapy and radiotherapy.[16] Such controlled trials are now commonplace practice and there must be hundreds of such procedures being carried out in the United Kingdom. They provide the definitive validation step in testing the efficacy of preventive and treatment regimens before they are introduced into practice.

For most therapeutic trials it is essential that there be a group of subjects receiving a different or no treatment, the attribution of subjects to one group or another being randomized. A control group should of course never include patients from whom a treatment of known benefit is withheld. The Statement by the Medical Research Council (1964) demands that the control group should 'receive the procedure previously accepted as the best'. The Declaration of Helsinki also states that 'in any medical study, every patient — including those of a control group, if any — should be assured of the best proven diagnostic and therapeutic method'. Both the MRC Statement and the Helsinki Code include additional provisions for the protection of the individual patient: 'It goes without question that any doctor taking part in such a collective trial is under an obligation to withdraw a patient from the trial, and to institute any treatment he considers necessary, should this, in his personal opinion, be in the better interests of his patient.' The Helsinki Declaration binds doctors with the words 'the health of my patient will be my first consideration'.

Patients should be made fully aware of the evidence concerning the treatments under evaluation before enrolling. Patients and investigators alike must be convinced that there is no satisfactory evidence to differentiate the effectiveness of one treatment over the other under test, or, over another treatment available outside the trial. Another ethical consideration is the assurance that sufficient testing has been undertaken *a priori* to ensure that any toxic or effects of the treatment is minimized. Every trial must be constantly modified for such effects, and the protocol must have well defined procedures for both reporting and analysing such effects.

Objections are sometimes raised about the way these procedures are carried out in man. The objections are mainly directed at (1) the use of the null hypothesis, (2) the double blind technique, (3) random allocation to treatments, and (4) the use of placebos. The main criticism is that controlled trials, and placebo trials in particular, deceive the patient and so infringe patient's rights as well as being ethically degrading to both parties.[17]

Placebos

It is generally recognized that the use of placebos is ethically justified when it is appropriate. It should be explained to the subject that he or she may not be receiving the treatment under investigation. There can be no deception if the subject is fully informed with respect to the nature of the protocol. On the other hand practices which require that those receiving placebos be led to believe that they are receiving a medication are deceptive, under such circumstances the patient is definitely wronged even when not harmed. Patients prefer honesty and candour to deception, no matter how well meaning. The working out of the exact wording of an explanation of the trial can highlight the ethical issues and avoid deception. It must be borne in mind that certain words can have a profound emotional impact and be easily misunderstood. Placebos must be used just as ethically and scientifically as any other part of the clinical trial.

Double-Blind Trials

Double-blind trials are those in which neither investigator nor subject knows which subjects have received the new treatment or which have received a conventional treatment or placebo. This procedure is an attempt to neutralize bias in the trial arising from either the doctor's attitude to the patient or the patient's attitude to the doctor and the medication given.

I asked Dr Peter Elwood if he would kindly explain as

simply as possible the reasons for the use of double-blind trials and placebos.

'The evaluation of a drug, or a treatment of any kind, necessitates a comparison of the effect of that drug and the effect of either another treatment, or more usually, no treatment. It is essential that neither the doctor nor the patient knows which treatment is being given, otherwise the expectations of one, or of both, may lead to biased estimates of benefit. This is fairly obvious if the outcome of treatment is an effect on symptoms, but it can also apply to other more complex outcomes. For example, in a trial of a drug which may reduce the incidence of heart attacks, such as aspirin or betablockers, some patients will be given the active drug and others, selected at random, will be given placebos, that is, a pill or capsule which looks and tastes identical to the active drug. If this last is not given then both patient and doctor will know whether or not an active drug is being taken by a particular patient. If a patient in such a trial gets a chest pain he is less likely to do anything about it if he knows he is taking an active drug than he will if he is not taking anything. Furthermore, the doctor conducting the trial is likely to be more easily persuaded that a heart attack has occurred, whatever the evidence he is evaluating, if he knows that a patient has not been taking the drug under investigation.

Hence the need for placebos. No one likes using placebos but they are essential in a well designed trial. The "informed consent" given by patients included in a trial is in response to a description of the trial and this will state that some patients will receive the drug under investigation and some will not. Neither the nature of the drug being tested, nor the fact that some will not get the drug, is concealed from any patient. In any case, the patients on placebo often seem to derive some psychological benefit from taking something. Often, at the end of a trial, patients will describe how the tablets have helped, and afterwards it will be found that some of these have been on a placebo. Furthermore, the surveillance of patients in a trial, both in order to measure beneficial effects and to detect harmful effects, is usually much closer than in a conventional therapeutic situation. Guidelines are always drawn up for a trial and if a patient deteriorates, or if certain undesirable side-effects develop, then the trial treatment is withdrawn and conventional care is instituted. It can be said, with confidence, that the standard of care of patients in placebo controlled trials is usually very high indeed.'

Volunteers

No pressure should ever be imposed upon a volunteer. Much research has been done in America on prisoners and servicemen, but in the United Kingdom they have not been deemed as suitable volunteers as they are open to much vulnerability; for example, loss of parole or early discharge, or loss of promotion, should they not volunteer. Although there may sometimes be need for assessment of new therapeutic measures to prevent miscarriage or to treat diseases of pregnancy, women of child bearing age or who are pregnant should seldom be used for early clinical studies of drugs. It is deemed unethical too for early clinical studies of drugs to be carried out with mortally ill patients.

The freedom to refuse to participate or to withdraw at any stage as participants is important where the subjects have any sort of dependent relationship to the investigator — students, laboratory technicians, for example. Payment to volunteers can also influence the ethical situation on the system of 'rewards'. Discussing this, Professor O. L. Wade commented:

'Any system of reward as a patient or a volunteer who participates in experimental work must be such that there can be no question of subjects being bribed to submit to unreasonable hazards. On the other hand it is unreasonable to ask subjects to give up a whole day and a night to take part in a pharmaco-kinetic study of a drug without offering some compensation. Similarly it is highly desirable that those who plan and conduct clinical research should not have their judgement in any way perverted by monetary reward or expectation of professional advancement.'

It is the responsibility of an ethics review committee to determine whether the level of remuneration offered is within reasonable limits. An immense amount of goodwill exists in healthy lay people to offer themselves as volunteers, but every project to be undertaken should go to an ethics committee first.

Individual Versus Society

Is there a conflict between individual rights and the rights of society? How far can we ask one human being to take part in trials which may not benefit himself, or, perhaps, even the present generation? These were some of the questions I put to a small group of philosophers, physicians, and a medical student assembled in the Fellows Lounge, Green College, Oxford. Michael Lockwood, a young philosopher, had strong views to express:

'The answer to the question is, Yes, there is a conflict. The arguments one sometimes hears from doctors to suggest that there's no conflict are, in my view, entirely specious. One argument that one hears constantly from doctors goes something like this: Assume you have two forms of treatment and you want to tell which is the better. (One form of treatment may be no treatment — doing nothing, or merely administering a placebo.) Now either you know which form of treatment is better or you don't. If you know which one is the better then of course there is no need to run a clinical trial. But if, on the other hand, you don't know which is better, then it's perfectly ethical to choose randomly, in the case of any particular patient, which form of treatment he receives. That argument, as I say, is specious. And the reason it's specious is that it merely contrasts complete agnosticism with the state of complete knowledge, totally ignoring the points in between. The case where there's a conflict is where either the doctor is pretty sure that one form of treatment is superior, but wants to establish conclusively whether that is the case, or where the doctor is quite sure himself that one form of treatment is superior, but realizes that a nice statistically convincing trial is necessary if he is going to convince his colleagues. In either of those cases, if he carries out a clinical trial, it's just inevitable that he is going, in the case of some of the patients, to be administering a form of treatment which, in his judgement, is probably inferior. That seems to me to be an inescapable conflict. What one should do about the conflict is a very difficult issue. But that such a conflict exists is, to me, as clear as daylight.'

Mrs Gill Lockwood, a clinical medical student, took her husband's comments one stage further:

'The mere fact that such a conflict exists doesn't necessarily end the argument there. We could take it further along consequentialist lines. Even if there is a conflict we may still be entitled to weigh benefit to society against sub-optimal treatment for a few patients and come down in favour of a trial. Austin Bradford Hill makes that point quite clearly in one of his very influential articles in medical ethics where he says that the extent to which we are prepared to countenence a randomized clinical trial may often depend on the severity of the complaint that we are dealing with and the likelihood of the efficacy of the treatment we can offer. Where we have people coming into contact with the common cold, it might be quite acceptable to give some of them sugar-pills and some of them the latest wonder-drug, simply to see if it really works. Where, on the other hand, we have people at no risk of getting a particular disease, to give some of them a placebo in order to convince ourselves that the other treatment is better than nothing seems unacceptable. And between those two extreme cases we seem to have a whole spectrum of severity of disease plus efficacy of treatment.'

Dr Iain Chalmers, Director of the National Perinatal Epidemiology Unit at the Radcliffe Infirmary, Oxford, stated that his concern was

'to protect the individuals receiving interventions of whatever sort from the unpredicted adverse affects of those interventions. Clinical trials protect individuals at both a societal level (through the knowledge gained from experiments on other people) and as current patients too.'

There are two areas, according to Professor Duncan Vere, in which one may ask someone to participate:

'One, with full and open knowledge, to consent as an individual, or helped by relatives or a "subject's friend", given that the risks are trivial or extremely rare; and two, to make a real sacrifice, given full and open explanation, provided that peer review accepts the value and right-ness of the invitation — that is, it would seem wrong to make sacrifice impossible in the medical field.'

Professor Richens saw the issues as extremely difficult:

'It involves us particularly when we do normal volunteer experiments, which we do a lot in this department. Our practice is to have a panel of medical students whom we know are willing to volunteer. When we have a clinical trial coming up of a drug we would ask these students to take part. They are perfectly fit and healthy and so they, themselves, are going to get no benefit whatsoever apart from financial.'

As the Professor had made mention of finance, I asked about fees for volunteers:

'We agree upon a fee at the beginning. We have guide-lines within the Medical School as to how much we should be paying volunteers. We therefore offer that as a fee for students who are prepared to come along and take part in the trials, but there is no benefit to them and there is of course risk. Now it may be very small. If we have designed our trials right then the risk should be minimal, but there is always a risk in giving a new drug to anyone. I've always asked myself whether any volun-teer should be expected to take drugs or whether the whole business is completely unethical. The reason we do it is that the Committee on the Safety of Medicine demands toxicology, not just in animals but also in clin-ical studies as well. So these volunteer experiments are demanded by drug companies because the CSM in turn demands it of them. But I just wonder whether anybody is entitled to ask another perfectly healthy person to take a risk on behalf of society or of patients who have a disease. Volunteers perhaps don't think about that too much. But is giving money for that sort of risk ethical? I don't know of any answer. We do it, but from time to time it bothers me. In our present state of medical science there is no alternative for animal and human experiments'.

Confidentiality

Another recurring ethical problem is the right to privacy in experimentation with human subjects. The right of privacy is fundamental to the dignity and freedom of a human person. Intimate personal data and information, clinical records, research papers and computerized storage should not be made available to other researchers without prior consent of the patient or subject involved. Whenever it is possible anonymity should be incorporated into all research and experimentation and there should be no misuse of what is privileged and private information. All personal identification should be destroyed as soon as possible.

There is at present much public concern about the use of computers, data banks and institutional records, and the strictest rules and regulations governing their protection of confidentiality are necessary. Whenever possible all such information should be coded in order to provide the strictest security within the system.

Compensation

Both subject and investigator should be protected in the event of injury which may be incurred during research procedures, for despite the exercise of the highest degree of skill and care and competence by the investigator injury may occur. On the one hand the patient is in justice entitled to compensation for injury or disability he may have suffered in experiments designed to benefit others. On the other the investigator has also the right to be protected against legal action or damage to his medical reputation from alleged or actual injury to the patient in valid experimental situations.

The present legal position appears to be somewhat unsatisfactory. It states that should an accident occur, the individual who suffers the injury is entitled to compensation only if negligence can be shown on the part of the research worker or members of his team. In the absence of negligence the only other means by which a research subject or his dependant might receive compensation would be by applying for an ex gratia payment from the sponsor of the research or the researcher's employing authority. Dr Robert Mahler stressed the importance of the subject of compensation and remarked on the present unsatisfactory legal situation:

> 'I personally think that there should be a fund out of which payment should be made to compensate for damage ensuing unexpectedly and not through negligence on anyone's part. Many of the drug firms are prepared to help here. It's very important that people do negotiate this beforehand.'

The Royal Commission on Civil Liability and Compensation for Personal Injury Report, (London: HMSO: March 1978: Cmnd 7054), known as the Pearson Report, states that the basis for compensation for prescribed drugs should be that of strict liability. Cause and effect have to be proved, but negligence is not an issue. In paragraph 1341 of the Report there is an important recommendation relating to injury incurred by a volunteer: 'Any volunteer for medical research or clinical trials who suffers severe damage as a result should have a course of action on the basis of strict liability against the authority to which he has consented to make himself available.'

The Ciba Foundation Study Group (1980) on the above Report considered the three possible ways of providing compensation: (1) negligence, (2) strict liability, and (3) a 'no fault' scheme. As stated, negligence is the basis of the present law of compensation for accidents in medical research: 'In order to receive compensation the injured person must show a failure to take reasonable care or to exercise reasonable skill on the part of someone involved in the research.' The injured person has to prove negligence. 'If the accident occurred without negligence on anyone's part, or if it resulted from an error of judgement that anyone could have made despite the use of reasonable care and skill, no compensation will be legally possible'(p. 4).

The Pearson Commission considered liability based on negligence to be unsatisfactory, and stated that they 'think that it is wrong that a person who exposes himself to some medical risk in the interest of the community should have to rely on ex gratia compensation in the event of injury' (para 1341).

Strict liability may be defined as 'liability, irrespective of negligence of the defendant or of someone for whom he is responsible, based solely on proof that he caused the injury of which the claim is made', and the claimant 'must seek redress through the courts against a named defendant, and the burden of proof of causation falls upon the claimant'.

The term 'no fault' which was used by the Royal Commission (Pearson Report 1978) refers to 'compensation which is obtainable without proving fault and is provided outside the tort system. No-fault compensation is a system of obtaining payment from a fund instead of proceeding against the person responsible for the injury' (Pearson Report, paragraph 34). Compensation paid under these circumstances would be very much akin to an insurance system.

The Ciba Study Group in summing up its recommendations conclude 'that a no-fault scheme would provide the most satisfactory means for compensating participants (or their relatives) for injuries received as a consequence of medical research', and suggests that 'a fund should be established, administered by a board, to provide compensation on a no-fault basis, to which those injured (or their dependants) could make direct application' (p. 9).

Doctor-Patient Relationship

Some doctors suggest that it is unreasonable to expect the physician to adopt a dual role as physician/investigator, that is, one for the care of the patient, the other for the experiment. The relationship can so easily become violated for it is difficult for any one doctor to assume the divided responsibilities of both 'scientist' and 'helper'. The needs of the doctor can very well be projected and influence patient relationship. Each is likely to be affected by subjective elements, as Balint (1964) showed in his study of *The Doctor, his Patient and the Illness* (Pitman Medical, London, 1964). Again the doctor himself can become far too fascinated and intrigued with the disease so that his relationship with the patient becomes fragmented and the loyalties of the doctor/patient relationship and those of research clash.

Who obtains consent from the patient and how is this affected by the relationship between them? Does the dual role of physician/investigator create any psychological and emotional as well as practical problems? Professor Wade again explained to me how he resolved these possible difficulties:

> 'It is because one is worried about the possibility that my interest in research may make me less concerned about my patient that I turn to one of my colleagues who is not involved in this study and say, Look, is this study all right? I personally have never felt that any of the studies I have done has in any way reduced my concern or my care for the individual patient or in any way interfered with the human dignity of my patient.'

The problem is somewhat eased when investigator and physician are different people, the one primarily interested in the scientific problem, the other in the medical care and welfare of the patient. Should a team approach be involved in the research programme there must be a leader who is prepared to assume full responsibility. As one physician aptly described the dilemma: 'The patient knows how he feels, but does not know what he has got; the doctor knows what the patient has got, but does not know how he feels!' The doctor/patient relationship soon becomes violated should the investigation carried out confer little or no conceivable benefit to the patient, and there must be certainty in the doctor's mind that the expected benefit of a particular medical or surgical procedure will outweigh the estimated risk. The welfare of the patient is always the prime and overriding consideration.

Ethical Committees

It was inevitable that a certain degree of abuse came about over the years in the whole sphere of experimentation, and it was H. K. Beecher (1966) in the USA, and M. H. Pappworth (1967) in England[18] who drew the public's attention in the mid-1960s to undesirable and unnecessary experiments which had been performed. To allay a general critical atmosphere the Royal College of Physicians of London issued later a statement in 1973: *Supervision of the Ethics of Clinical Research Investigations in Institutions*, and arising from these recommendations ethical committees or research ethical committees came to be set up.

Such committees to which all research projects are to be submitted are now firmly established in the majority of, if not all, teaching hospitals as well as many of the other large hospitals in which research programmes are carried out. The purpose of these committees is to act as a safeguard to all those patients and healthy volunteers who participate in research and to ensure a reasonable ethical standard in human experimentation programmes. As the Royal College Report outlines: 'The object of ethical committees is to safeguard patients, healthy volunteers and the reputation of the profession and its institutions in matters of clinical research investigations . . . To function efficiently ethical committees should be small and they must not be constituted as to cause an unreasonable hindrance to the advancement of medical knowledge.'

It was also recommended that in addition to the membership of experienced clinicians with the knowledge and experience of clinical research there should be a lay member. (The Health Authorities were asked in DHSS Circular: HSC (15) 153 to consider appointing a lay member of a health council to serve on its ethical committees.) The Council of the British Medical Association has recently approved recommendations from its Central Ethical Committee for a change in the composition of ethical review committees.[19] Recent proposals for a model constitution of these committees include the appointment of:

(1) two senior hospital doctors, nominated by medical executive committee,

(2) one junior hospital doctor, nominated by the appropriate junior medical committee,

(3) two general practitioners, nominated by the local medical committee staff, with local RCGP (Royal College of General Practitioners) faculty approval,

(4) one representative of community medicine, nominated by the appropriate community medicine staff,

(5) one nurse, and

(6) one lay member.

A research worker would find it extremely difficult to be supported by financial grants from the Medical Research Council or any other grant-aiding organization unless his research project had first been approved by his research ethics committee, and no reputable medical or scientific journal in the United Kingdom is prepared to publish any research papers unless they too have been satisfactorily considered and sanctioned by an REC.

What methodology then, if any, should be used in reaching judgements about which research projects are ethical? Who is qualified to review the performance of ethical committees? Dr John Scanlon answered the first question very fully for me:

'First, will the experiment answer the question asked? Second, are subjects exposed to undue risk to achieve the answer? Third, is coercion or unfair motivation a factor? Can subjects remove themselves? Is all necessary information available to them to make a rational choice? Fourth, is (or will) the experiment's course be appropriately monitored? Will adverse reactions be appropriately handled? Will the experimental data be available to subjects?'

I also discussed these questions with Dr William Silverman when we met at Helen House, Oxford. He placed much emphasis on the responsibility of the community:

'My own feeling is that groups representing the community should make final judgements in these matters. Unlike preclinical research (which thrives best when it is free-ranging) bedside studies should be sharply goal-directed and the goals must not be defined solely by physicians. There is a strong public interest in clinical studies because consequences extend well beyond immediate effects seen in individual patients. I think the balance of interests is protected when physician-researchers act only in an advisory role — provide technical details about the project and make arguments about expected gains for enrolled patients and for the public as a whole.'

Professor Charles George saw the peer system playing a major role in such decision-making:

'The performance of ethical committees should presumably be reviewed from time to time. In particular, the committee itself should endeavour to keep itself informed of any problems which may have arisen. They may also wish to "police" the obtaining of informed consent. Finally, there may be a place for a "super" peer system consisting of people with considerable experience with the operation of such committees drawn from other health districts.'

Ethical committees themselves are sufficient, according to Professor Duncan Vere, provided that they

'include lay membership, informed expertise, and have a checklisting procedure to prevent omission of significant questions. The performance depends largely upon the chairman, especially whether he or she is resolute in centring the business upon the patient's interests.'

At Northwick Park Hospital I spoke not only with Dr Robert Mahler but also with Dr Michael Denham. I found they had an excellent system to deal with these rather difficult issues. Dr Mahler explained it to me:

'I think we are the only hospital in the country that has two ethical committees. One is a Scientific Advisory Committee which assesses what one might term the value of the experiment; if it's properly designed, for example; what is likely to be achieved; the possible risks which may be involved, or any other hazards that may arise; and to assess the potential value of the experiment so that its aim is clearly outlined and defined. They may well say, What you are trying to achieve is hardly worth the doing, or, It is a valuable piece of research and on scientific grounds we think it is well worth pursuing. We have the Scientific Advisory Committee as well as the Ethical Committee because it is unethical to carry out an experiment on anyone if the science is not right. There is then no need to consider the ethical issues — it is just unethical to proceed. If they are right, then the main Ethical Committee, which includes lay persons, a nurse, general practitioner and hospital staff, assesses the ethical issues involved.'

Dr Michael Denham outlined the composition of the Scientific Committee and emphasized how supportive its screening methods proved to be:

'The Scientific Advisory Group consists of a chairman and three members of the scientific staff of the Clinical Research Centre, nominated by the Director. One of the three is always a statistician. One of the other members is an expert in radioisotopes and his knowledge has proved most valuable. The Group sees all projects before they are submitted to the Ethical Committee to ensure that the proposals are clearly set out, have a clearly defined, reasonably attainable objective and that the design methods are appropriate to achieve that objective. The Group meets monthly about two weeks before the Ethical Committee meets, so that there is usually very little hold up in consideration of submitted projects. If there is a need for rapid action, a project can be seen within a few days by members of the Advisory Group and it can then be passed to the Chairman of the Ethical Committee for his action.'

Ethical Considerations
By its very definition an experiment involves risk or choice, for it is an attempt to discover something which is unknown. It is because of this element of chance that ethics play such an important part in experiments with human subjects. For example, any clinical research which is not directly for the

benefit of the patient on whom it is performed raises a number of ethical problems, and brings to the forefront the conflict between individual and social good. Is it right to expose some individuals to risk for the positive benefit of others? Is it permissible to compromise the doctor/patient relationship by allowing it to be used for purposes other than healing?

Dr Douglas J. Whalan (1975) explained the problem as follows: 'We can posit extremes. On the one hand, the human body must not be regarded as a mine to be quarried for tissues and organs. Humans should not be regarded as commodities made up of useful spare parts and more than ninety per cent water; on the other hand, society can demand that certain medical procedures be undertaken for the good of society. Vaccination is an example, even although vaccination may in some cases involve a risk of encephalitis. Society demands this sacrifice by individuals; but how much can society demand? . . . The middle way must be discovered between the good of the general community and the complete integrity of private rights.'[20]

Has the patient a sense of duty or responsibility to co-operate in research? I found here a diversity of opinion. The majority of doctors thought that patients do have a sense of duty but this must not be exploited in any way. As we have already seen, medical progress depends upon some patients being prepared to contribute to the common good by voluntarily serving as experimental subjects.

> 'We all expect advances to take place in medicine', responded Professor Richens, 'whether it is in treatment or investigation, and patients must have a sense of responsibility once they have been informed about the nature of the problem. I think they should be expected to have some degree of understanding, that the only way in which advances take place is by participation of people like themselves — with diseases. There is no other way of testing new advances, particularly so in the drug field because all the animal work which goes on does not necessarily predict what will happen when the drug goes into man, and the only way of looking at the therapeutic effect in a disease is to use the drug in that disease.'

Dr Peter Elwood was of the same mind in his reply:

> 'I think patients do have a responsibility. I do not think one can argue too forcibly, but patients are benefiting from medical progress made because of the co-operation of other patients in the past. I feel therefore there is some sense of responsibility, but I would not urge it too strongly. If we are prepared to benefit from the work of others, then we in turn should be willing to contribute.'

Professor Duncan Vere too had no doubt:

> 'There is an ethical onus on patients to assist research; at times refusal is entirely understandable when seen against the patient's perceived discomfort or level of current information, but some refusals do seem to indicate a degree of self-centredness or misunderstanding. Modern medicine could not have attained its level of success without knowledge gained from innumerable experiments; it is all to easy to take this for granted and forget the contributions made by many volunteers who took part in those studies.'

A caveat came from Professor William Weil:

> 'As a matter of importance in patient care it is essential that the patient understand that his physician's concerns and care, and his overall treatment will in no way be altered if he chooses not to take part in research. This is critical for a freely given informed consent.'

It is evident that medical progress can only be made by means of experimentation; yet any risk, no matter how small, to the patient cannot be justified. Ethical committees must be highly responsible bodies to ensure not only the scientific validity of research projects submitted to them but also the maintenance of the highest ethical principles. Poorly designed studies are quite unethical, and it is the work of these committees to see that 'informed' or 'true' consent, the minimum risks outweighed by possible benefits, are stringently observed, and all investigations submitted to the most vigorous ethical scrutiny and self-discipline. A maxim of Pappworth's should always be kept in mind: 'An experiment is ethical or not at its inception, and does not become so post hoc because it achieved some measure of success.'[21] Or as it was put to me by Peter Elwood: 'No trial is better than a bad trial.'

The interest of the patient must always come first, and the Declaration of Geneva of the World Medical Association binds the doctor with the words, 'The health of my patient will be my first consideration.' Research can so easily become an end in itself — research *on* the patient rather than research *for* the patient. No human being should be 'used' for the sole purpose of acquiring medical knowledge in the abstract. Patients are not 'teaching material' to be divested of all the elements that make man human and uniquely a person, and there must be a stand against all processes which dehumanize and depersonalize.

Essential as such experimentation might be, personal rights — privacy, dignity, freedom and informed consent — must not be sacrificed. Man is not a test-tube obeying the laws of physics and chemistry, but a spiritual being. In this respect it is worth recalling two important dicta of that great humanitarian and scientist of a century or more ago, Claude Bernard, the father of experimental medicine: 'The principle of medical morality consists, then, in never performing on man an experiment which can be harmful to him in any degree whatsoever, though the results may be of great interest to science — that is, of benefit to save the health of others . . . Among the experiments that may be tried on man, those that may do good are obligatory.'[22] Simplistic as such an approach may appear to be in today's exciting scientific world the principles themselves are well worth bearing in mind.

Impartial and essential as codes of practice may be, ultimately the overall standards of conduct in the whole field of human experimentation must depend on the right ethical standards of all those investigators and research workers who are engaged in furthering scientific and medical studies. They can be no substitute for the basic trust and confidence between doctor and patient.

Who is to define the ethical and moral rights and obligations of all those who are involved — medical, paramedical, patients? The majority of the doctors agreed that it was the responsibility of society, or, to be more specific, *all* of the above mentioned and more! Dr John Scanlon suggested:

> 'A committee of each group's peers, conveniently defined as a human subjects committee, composed of scientists, health care providers, religious and legal experts plus consumers.'

Professor Duncan Vere explained that to his way of thinking:

> 'There is no such thing as "essential rights" — there are *agreed* rights. For example, legal rights, rights accepted by the United Nations or WHO, or rights determined by religious presuppositions — for Christians and for Jews, the right of innocent lives to safeguard. Hence rights are "defined" by societal agreement. Duties are another matter. I may feel a duty far beyond what society may require of me, hence I have defined duties determined by law, by employers, by tutors, etc., etc., but I may resolve to go beyond them. With regard to research it seems wise for agreed rights and safeguards to be *proposed* by doctors and by patients, and agreed by society at large. Much expertise is required to propose them — hence local ethics committees.'

It is encouraging to note a suggested modification to the Helsinki Code made at the International Conference on Human Experimentation at Bossey 1969, and published in the WCC Report, *Experiments with Man* (World Council Studies No 6), p. 27. 'Medical Schools, Universities and teachers should ensure that every future doctor and related research worker should be made familiar with the ethics of experimentation including the factors which influence its decision making progress.' Where a right and proper balance of ethical control is maintained patients can be fully protected and essential medical research continue to flourish.

The author wishes to acknowledge his gratitude to Owen L. Wade, Dean of the Faculty of Medicine and Dentistry, Professor of Therapeutics and Clinical Pharmacology, University of Birmingham, for commenting upon and reading through the original draft of this chapter for medical accuracy.

2
Organ Transplantation

Tissue grafting, skin, blood vessel, bone, and cornea, has now been regularly performed for many years. Organ transplantation on the other hand may be said to have begun when the first kidney was successfully transplanted in the mid-1950s by Murray, Merrill and Harrison (1954) at the Peter Bent Brigham Hospital, Boston, USA, from a healthy twin into the other twin who was suffering from renal failure.[1] In the early 1960s the era of modern organ grafting commenced, with the use of imuran and corticosteroids for kidney grafting, and when Calne (1960) proved the efficacy of such drugs the scene was set in the UK for the modern era of kidney transplantation.[2] In 1967 the MRC (Medical Research Council) advised the Department of Health that the transplantation of kidneys had passed the stage of pure research.

Many thousands of kidneys had been successfully transplanted when the first human heartgraft was performed by Professor Christiaan Barnard at the Groote Schuur Hospital, Cape Town, on 31 December 1967.[3] This was only made possible by the pioneering experimental work of Professor Shumway in Stanford, California, who now has by far the largest series of successful heart transplants.

In the following year Mr Donald Ross performed the first British heart transplant at the National Heart Hospital, London. This was followed by a spate of such operations which were carried out by various surgical teams in many different countries, the majority of which were failures.

Public controversy was aroused and surgeons discouraged by the obvious lack of success. Many people were aghast at the whole idea of heart transplantation, regarding the heart as the inviolate seat of the emotions. There was a lull while techniques were perfected and immuno-suppressive drugs developed, and surgical teams in the UK more or less abandoned such operations by the year 1970. In 1978/79 two surgeons, Mr Terence English at Papworth Hospital, near

Cambridge, and Mr Magdi Yacoub at Harefield Hospital, Middlesex, recommenced heart-transplants and since then approximately two hundred such operations have been performed at these two main centres in Britain. Over the past decade there lingered a sense of taboo, prejudice and superstition among not a few people about the concept of transplanting organs such as the kidneys, lungs, liver and heart — live organs from dead people. But organ transplantation seems now to be approved by the majority of people in the United Kingdom and most seem prepared to consent for their organs to be removed after death and for their relatives' kidneys to be transplanted after death.

Donors

Over the years considerable publicity has been given to the need for donors. The Code of Practice (i.e. *Cadaveric Organs for Transplantation*: 1983) states that: 'Patients who may become suitable donors after death are those who have suffered severe and irreversible brain damage. Such patients will be dependent on artificial ventilation or expected shortly to become so . . . It is not always easy to recognize whether a patient would be considered a suitable donor should he die. For example, patients who have had a sudden irreversible cardio-respiratory arrest (for example, myocardial infarction) or those in the so-called "brought in dead" category are unlikely to be suitable as organ donors'.[4] Although large numbers of patients die in hospital whose organs are suitable for transplantation, and opinion polls indicate that the general public are in favour of organ transplantation, there is still a great shortage of donor supply and the majority of the thirty main transplant centres are working at well below their potential capacity and performing fewer than half the number of operations for which they were designed. There seems more than enough potential donors available in particular cases of cerebral trauma and haemorrhage, both of which conditions are very often the result of injuries sustained in road and other accidents. Doctors themselves seem reluctant to initiate the process and in many instances one finds that it is the next of kin or relatives of the deceased who are more forthcoming. What are some of the factors responsible for the shortage of organs?

'The two main factors responsible for the shortage of organs for transplantation,' commented Professor Peter Morris, 'are firstly, public concern, and secondly, dislike by doctors in getting involved in what can be a rather distressing as well as time-consuming process of talking to relatives about the possibility of providing organs at the same time as they have to tell the relatives that the patient is dead.'

The position was spelt out in practical terms by Mr P. J. Wilson:

'(1) Most important, *medical* unsuitability of the possible donor — for example, because of age, cardiovascular or other major system disease, infection, cancer, unfavourable immune status. (2) Next most important, reluctance or aversion or indifference or poor organization of the doctor's medical men. (3) Next, absence of consent by next of kin; more rarely, legal objection by coroner or others — for example, in the case of unlawful killing, murder, assault. (4) Organizational obstacles — for example, non-availability of an operating theatre, or of transplant team personnel, at the optimum time for the surgical process of harvesting.'

The medical profession's ambivalence about transplantation as a whole was also raised by Dr Victor Parsons. Another reason he gave was:

'The criteria for brain death have undergone some revisions which have made it perhaps even more complicated to get permission to remove organs, in that teams of people have to see the patient twice in two days to make quite sure the patient's brain is dead. This, in one sense, causes delay, and when there is pressure on beds in intensive care units people would rather not bother to go through this procedure, which has been tightened up, quite rightly I think, to assure the public that everything has been done for the particular patient . . . It's a very good example of Titmus' "gift relationship" — it is really a gift which is involving them, and this is something where you just have to ask them to go that extra mile and think of other patients whom they don't see.'

That the major factor, 'without a shadow of doubt, is the medical profession', was a point reiterated by Mr Michael Bewick, who commented on

'their general unawareness of the need. They know it intellectually, but when they see it emotionally in front of them they don't actually think about it.'

Mr Bewick went on to praise and applaud the attitude of the general public:

'I think the public of this country are magnificent — they really are. You've only got to go and see relatives when they've got their nearest and dearest dying, and less than five per cent say "No". We basically are very socially aware of each other's needs. It's usually the parents of little children. They say, "You know John is dying. Have you thought about using his kidneys, doctor?"'

Professor Bryan Jennett (1975) also recognizes that the public are ahead of the profession and often initiate the use of their relatives' kidneys for transplantation purposes when the doctors had not thought about it. Many of the doctors caring for potential donors feel insecure and do not wish to make any decision that might be questioned from the point of view of the law or on ethical grounds.[5]

The evidence seems to prove that only about one brain dead patient in ten is offered as a donor.

A Gallup Poll[6] on kidney donors (4–9 March 1981) reported the following results on people's attitudes to donation of organs for transplantation:

1011 People Questioned

Q.1. Would you agree to donate your kidneys for transplantation after your death?
Yes   59%   No   27%   Don't know 14%

Q.2. Are you a kidney donor?
Yes   16%   No   84%

Q.3. Do you carry a kidney donor card?
    Yes   18%   No   82%

Q.4. After recent publicity (the BBC Panorama programme
    of 13 October, 1980) are you *more* or *less* inclined to
    donate your kidneys?
    More   12%   Less   16%   Unaffected 72%

The number of willing kidney donors is almost precisely the
same as in July 1980, when the Gallup survey was last carried
out. Many units have appointed nurses or lay persons as
co-ordinators with responsibility for providing an information
and education service.

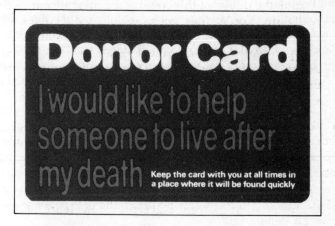

Donor Card
I would like to help someone to live after my death

Keep the card with you at all times in a place where it will be found quickly

I request that after my death

*(a) my *kidneys. *eyes. *heart. *liver. *pancreas be used
    for transplantation; or
*(b) any part of my body be used for the treatment of others
*(delete if not applicable)

Signature   Date

Full name (block capitals)

In the event of my death. if possible contact:

Name   Telephone

It is estimated that about four million people have signed donor cards but an informal survey carried out by the co-ordinators at the Department of Health's transplant co-ordination headquarters showed that only eight out of 2,000 donors were card holders, and they did not all have their cards on them at death. One-third of donors are accident victims who, when entering casualty units, are without their donor cards. The whole concept of donor cards therefore relies heavily on public opinion and awareness.

There was at one time a degree of uncertainty about the legal validity of the kidney donor card produced by the Department of Health and Social Security. For example, could a person in charge of the body of the deceased authorize the removal of organs without enquiring whether the next of kin objected beforehand? Fortunately the Department issued a Guidance Circular (1975)[7] which stated that the card is 'a written expression of his wishes in accordance with section 1 (1) of the (Human Tissue) Act', and 'the fact that the deceased was carrying a card would be strong evidence that the request has not been withdrawn.' It further stated that when the Health Authority is 'the person lawfully in posses-sion of the body, the deceased has signed such an authoriz-ation, and the relatives subsequently ask for the return of the body, this action does not revoke the authorization — which continues to be legally effective.' The donor card is now officially recognized as legally acceptable evidence of a per-son's wish for his organs to be removed after death.

I discussed the issue of donor cards with Dr Victor Parsons at King's College Hospital, and Mr Michael Bewick in his office on the top floor of the tower block of Guy's Hospital, London. Dr Parsons explained that the card

> 'is an indication to the relatives that this is the person's wishes; but the relatives can still overrule this, and there's no mandate to ignore the relatives.'

There would be few surgeons I assumed who would over-ride the family's wishes regardless of whether the patient had a card or not.

> 'Exactly', Dr Parsons affirmed. 'I think some people find it hard to bear. There is still something about the human

body that people wish to preserve *in toto*, despite whatever has happened to it.'

Mr Michael Bewick stated:

'We are specifically recommended by DHSS even if we find a donor card, to ask the relatives, just to be certain. There is only one instance where I've found the donor card, seen the relatives and they've said "No".'

The Human Tissue Act (1961)

This Act (see Appendix II p. 210) governs the obtaining of donor material, but was devised before the recent great advances in surgical techniques in transplant operations and is somewhat ambiguous in some of its provisions, being a mixture of 'contracting in' and 'contracting out' systems. There is, for example, no special consideration in the Act for the needs of transplant surgery which obviously require that organs be removed without delay. Section 1(1) is a 'contracting in' provision, and states: 'If any person, either in writing at any time or orally in the presence of two or more witnesses during his last illness, has expressed a request that his body or any specified part of his body be used after his death for therapeutic purposes or for purposes of medical education or research, the person lawfully in possession of his body after his death may, unless he had reason to believe that the request was subsequently withdrawn, authorize the removal from the body of any part or, as the case may be, the specified part, for use in accordance with the request.'

Section 1(2) is in part a 'contracting out' provision, but it also enables the next of kin or relatives to veto the removal of organs, where the deceased did not request (in the manner specified in Section 1(1)) that his organs be so used. It states: 'Without prejudice to the foregoing subsection, the person lawfully in possession of the body of a deceased person may authorize the removal of any part from the body for use for the said purpose if, having made such reasonable enquiry as may be practicable, he has no reason to believe:

(a) that the deceased had expressed an objection to his body being so dealt with after his death, and had not withdrawn it; or

(b) that the surviving spouse or any surviving relative of
the deceased objects to the body being so dealt with.'

Although the intention might be clear, the conditions are
somewhat opaque. Difficulties have arisen regarding the
identity of the person '*in possession of the body*', and the meaning
of the term '*reasonable enquiry*'. The Guidance Circular to NHS
Authorities (DHSS 1975) referred to above states that the
Authority is in possession legally of the body until such time
as the executors, or whoever is under the legal duty to dispose
of the body, have requested its custody. Again as the Authority is a 'blanket' term, it has to be presumed that an administrator or his deputy is the person in possession of the body.
Where the hospital (i.e. the Authority) is in lawful possession,
and the deceased was carrying an appropriately worded and
signed 'donor card' the case falls within Section 1 (2).

Even less easy to define is the extent of '*reasonable enquiries*'.
It is obvious that, as there is extreme urgency so far as time is
concerned, such enquiries cannot be anything like exhaustive.
In 1973, for example, one surgeon was faced with an agonizing dilemma. He removed the kidneys of a 17-year-old killed
in a road accident without permission of the youth's parents
who were abroad in Spain on holiday and could not be con-
tacted in time. The Department of Health and Social Security
stated that its own legal advice was that in the absence of
claims by next of kin a hospital is 'lawfully in possession' of a
patient when he dies. In this particular incident the parents
themselves would have opposed the removal of their son's
organs.

As Robert A. Sells (1979) put it: 'The man who drafted this
paragraph in the Act obviously assumed that 12 to 24 hours
could elapse after the death before allowing organ removal to
proceed, without the organs being damaged to the extent that
they would be useless for therapeutic, research or educational
purposes. In 1961, when the law was drafted, the need to
remove kidneys within 30 to 60 minutes after cardiac arrest
was not universally appreciated. The new need for speed has
focused on the necessity to define "reasonable" and "practicable", since these terms define the limits within which an
administrator must work if he is to allow the legal removal of

organs'.[8] Under the circumstances, what is normally done is that written consent is obtained, wherever possible, from the nearest available relative, rather than to delay in ensuring an absence of refusal from a range of relatives.

The DHSS Guidance Circular on the Human Tissue Act (1975) suggests that 'in most instances it will be sufficient to discuss the matter with any one relative who has been in close contact with the deceased, asking him his own views, the views of the deceased and also if he has any reason to believe that any other relative would be likely to object'. If the letter of the Act was strictly adhered to, a request by the deceased person during his lifetime for his organs to be used cannot be overruled by his next of kin or relatives. In actual practice it would be extremely unusual for a surgeon to proceed with organ removal in the face of objections from the family.

As obvious difficulties have sometimes arisen regarding the identity of the person 'in possession of the body', and the meaning of the phrase 'reasonable enquiry', should the Human Tissue Act 1961 be altered to clarify these legal issues? As the number of kidneys that are lost as a result of these factors is negligible doctors do not regard it as in any way a major issue. As one of them explained: 'There is no problem regarding the identity of the person "in possession of the body". A next of kin, or the medical director/medical superintendent of the hospital is responsible for the body. I have within my mind no doubt regarding "reasonable inquiry", but if there is any doubt at all, this is passed on to the benefit. In the majority of instances, the relatives are available, and more than "reasonable inquiry" is made.' Mr Robert Sells referred to the helpful DHSS Guidance Circular (1975) mentioned above, and gave a further interesting comment:

> 'Lawyers find the Act infuriating because of the above (i.e. the phrases mentioned in the question). Most doctors work within it happily, and while recognizing its quirks, are very reluctant to rock the boat, or allow it to be rocked!'

A delightful comment, too, came from Mr Peter Wilson:

> 'No, it is all right as it stands, I think — "the letter killeth . . .".'

Support for the 'status quo' also came from Dr Victor Parsons:

> 'I think it's very difficult to legislate as to what is "reasonable enquiry". If you made it very watertight you would probably lose a proportion of organs . . . if the inquiry necessitated a vast search for a family on holiday or for relatives that a patient hadn't seen for a long time. It's best left as it is at the moment.'

Contracting In — Contracting Out

It has already been noted that the first sub-section of the Human Tissue Act (see p.210) provides for what has become known as 'contracting-in' — i.e. the deceased either in writing at any time or orally in the presence of two or more witnesses during his last illness, has expressed a request 'that his organs be used for transplanting'. The second subdivision provides for the circumstances in which the deceased has not expressed any wish.

There have been several attempts to change the law so that a person's organs might be removed without his permission and also without asking the relatives if they object. This would mean that a person in charge of the body could assume that the patient would not object to his body being so dealt with, unless it could be shown that the patient had recorded his objection during his lifetime — i.e. the procedure known as 'contracting out'. The advice given in the DHSS Code of Practice (*Cadaveric Organs for Transplantation 1983*) is that 'if a patient who has died is not known to have requested (in the required manner) that his organs be removed for transplantation after his death, the designated person may only authorize removal if, having made such reasonable enquiry as may be practicable, he has no reason to believe:

(a) that the deceased had expressed an objection to his body being so dealt with after his death, and had not withdrawn it; or

(b) that the surviving spouse or any surviving relative of the deceased objects to the body being so dealt with' (p.8).

An Advisory Group on transplantation problems, (The MacLennan Report: 1969[9]), laid down the highest standards of ethical conduct for cadaveric organ transplantation. It favoured a sweeping change in the law by a majority of six to five, saying that surgeons could remove any dead man's organs (heart, liver or kidneys) unless that person had specifically contracted out (i.e. objected to it during his lifetime) — a practice already existing in some European countries (in Austria, Denmark and France, the law provides for 'a contracting out' system). Donors should not be transported between hospitals purely to facilitate transplantation. Public education and enrolment forms should be encouraged. It also advocated that transplant surgeons and nephrologists foster co-operation within the rest of the profession and thereby increase the referral notes of organ donors from district hospitals and neurological units.

Another important recommendation was that the doctor clinically responsible for the care of the potential donor would always be different from the doctor clinically responsible for a prospective recipient. The MacLennan Report also emphasized the need to separate the management of a seriously ill patient from consideration of organ donation before death had taken place. (This important factor was later to be reinforced by the Royal Colleges' document on 'Brain Death' (1976), which states that a consultant or his deputy, and one other doctor should make the decision to discontinue artificial ventilation.) All members agreed on the need for some legal changes to encourage a much greater supply of organs for transplant. The DHSS Code of Practice (1979) later considered that it was not necessary to change to a 'contracting out' procedure as the Human Tissue Act was partly a 'contracting in' and partly a 'contracting out' arrangement.

As both 'contracting in' and 'contracting out' schemes have distinct disadvantages, should patients who are suitable donors have their kidneys removed without consent as postulated in certain continental countries? The majority of doctors were adamant that kidneys should definitely not be removed without consent. As one surgeon put it: 'I feel that with education we should certainly be able to receive adequate kidneys for transplantation. About 2,000 patients die every year on respirators, and those kidneys should be used for transplantation. This would provide 4,000 kidneys altogether, a number adequate to meet all the requirements of the patients in England.' Professor Peter Morris stated categorically:

> 'Donors should not have their kidneys removed without the permission of relatives, if their own wishes are unknown.'

This was a viewpoint shared by many others. The general consensus of opinion was that there should always be consent, freely given; if not indicated by the donor before his death, then given by next of kin. Mr Robert Sells saw the Human Tissue Act 1961 as a compromise, being a two-tier system:

> 'But it works, and it seems as though the public feel that their rights are protected by it.'

'Contracting in', properly done, does not appear to have any major disadvantages. Dr Victor Parsons confessed to being ambivalent about both 'contracting in' and 'contracting out'. He felt:

> 'Whatever system you have it's difficult to monitor; and although one would prefer far more people to contract in by carrying cards, at the moment a 'contracting out' scheme would be, I think, a little more than the public would want to agree to.'

Mr Michael Bewick was also rather worried and uneasy about either scheme.

> 'The "contracting out" scheme is a bad scheme', he felt. 'The "contracting in" scheme is the safest one in terms of the right of the individual.'

He agreed with Dr Victor Parsons that the public would need further education before any change was contemplated. They are certainly not ready for a scheme to remove organs regardless, but

> 'we will have to work towards it', and he considered it had a distinct advantage in that 'the public, the relatives don't need to be further upset by the whole process.

"Johnny's dead" is bad enough, but "Johnny's dead,
and can I have his kidneys, his liver, or his heart?" —
well!'

There were others who more or less supported this viewpoint. 'After all, if a post-mortem has to be done the organs
will be removed anyhow', was a typical reaction. In 1968 the
Church of Scotland's General Assembly voted in favour of
allowing removal of kidneys without either the consent of the
deceased in his lifetime or of the next of kin after his death.
Such a radical proposal may not at present commend itself to
the general public.

An attempt was made in the House of Commons in February 1984 to persuade the Government to set up an inquiry on
changing the law but this was not successful. Instead the
Government launched a campaign to persuade ten million
volunteers to carry donor cards. Michael Bewick was more in
favour of a middle way where people could be asked for their
agreement to donation, perhaps on census forms, and the
replies computerized.

From an ethical point of view there is much to be said
against the 'contracting-out' procedure. An interesting comment was made by Canon G. R. Dunstan (1969)[10] on the two
options. After asserting that 'contracting out' could find
theological support (e.g. very high value of human life,
coupled with that of family solidarity, preserving to a family 'a
healthy father or mother, say, for a few more years'), he went
on to state: 'but theology would balance these considerations
with others, relevant to man's place in civil society, and to the
manner of his serving the common good. It might argue that
the principle of mutuality, of our being members one of
another, is best served, and so far as possible should be served,
by action arising from free consent; that it is better for men to
offer the use of what they have for the common advantage
than that it should be taken from them without their express
will; that *to give* is more blessed than *not to mind*'.

The Report of the British Transplantation Society (1975)[11]
recommends that a register be established listing name, date
of birth, and address of persons who wish their bodies to be
used for transplantation after their death, and of those who

object to such use of their bodies. Provided ready access to this information was assured, such a register would greatly facilitate the enquiry required by S.1. (2) (Human Tissue Act 1961). It would also safeguard the interests of those persons who do not wish their bodies to be used for transplantation after their death.

Each year in the United Kingdom there are approximately 3,000 patients suffering from chronic renal failure. There are two established medical treatments.

(1) Haemodialysis

This treatment necessitates the patient to be attached to an artificial kidney machine for about thirty hours a week. The machine has two main components — the artificial kidney (the dialyser) which effectively washes the patient's blood and frees it from poisons which accumulate. The other component is the preparation machine which prepared the fluid which runs through the dialyser and washes the blood. It also has the added advantage of a monitoring system which not only monitors the strength of the solution but also its temperature and the pressure of the patient's blood as it goes through the artificial kidney. Should anything go wrong an alarm will ring. Although the number of renal units have increased rapidly in Britain over the years, the problem of selection of patients is still acute in some areas.

Parsons and Lock (1980) circulated nephrologists in twenty-five renal units with the clinical and social details of forty patients with renal failure who had undergone treatment at King's College Hospital, London. The physicians were invited to select ten patients who were to be rejected for dialysis and asked to state the reasons for their selection. As a result of the enquiry there was seen to be substantial discrepancies between different units. Only a third of the patients would have been selected by all units and no patient was rejected by all units. There was a consensus of opinion however which found certain groups of patients more difficult to accept: those with severe mental illness, with infectious disease, or considerable physical handicap comprising widespread complications of simple ageing alone. The disturbing feature of the enquiry was 'the extent to which physicians' professional expertise and position of trust is being used to translate economic and political decisions into the selection of patients, without those presenting with renal disease, their relatives or the public necessarily being aware of this process'. The Medical Services Study Group (The Clarke Report, 1981) also clearly shows the variation in the 'mix' of criteria for selection. Such major differences seem to reflect the variable resources allocated to chronic renal failure. There is also obvious geographical inequality.

A further complication is due to the fact that a patient's response to treatment cannot be reliably predicted. Clinical experience may help in making the assessment for treatment but, as Knapp (1982) shows, 'when treatment is provided for patients with an apparently poor prognosis surprisingly often those expected to fare badly may do well. There are, in fact, few objective measurements to predict the response to treatment. A trial of treatment is often the only reliable way of evaluating the physical and psychological suitability of patients, but stopping treatment once started is obvious to the patient and to the observer and is difficult for all concerned. There is no obvious answer to this dilemma.'

In view of such a mixture of criteria there seems evidence for more lay opinion to be sought where decisions are to be made on other than medical guidelines. Fox (1981) makes mention of lay help to aid decision-making in the USA, and Kennedy (1981) highlighted concern about the way doctors as a profession keep decision-making processes to themselves, and act as judge and jury. A number of the initial dialysis units originally had lay and medical committees through which the claims of potential patients were filtered. Such a procedure would spread the load of responsibility. At present a variety of conditions seem to control the definition of who is 'suitable' for selection.[12] The need seems to be not for more dialysis machines ('kidney machines') but for renal units and more trained personnel. Ideally all patients who are likely to benefit from such treatment should be accepted for it.

(2) Renal Transplantation

Most patients are only too pleased to be alive for the first few years on a kidney machine but the restrictions are irksome and the majority wish for kidney transplantation, which has now become an accepted therapy for terminal renal failure and offers an indisputable superior quality of life. It also restores the ability for women to conceive and to bear children, which is important to the younger woman. Mobility and freedom from the two or three times a week dialysis sessions is also another distinct advantage. Renal transplantation differs from other organ transplantation in so far as patients with renal failure can be maintained on haemodialysis or continuous ambulatory peritoneal dialysis (CAPD) whilst awaiting a transplant, or after rejecting a transplanted kidney. CAPD involves a plastic tube being inserted into the peritoneal cavity and then let run out, the cycle being repeated for 48 hours every three or four days. It is now in use in over eighty per cent of UK renal centres. It is a popular therapy which has been developed over the past two or three years. Patients can be trained to use it at home, and it has provided treatment for a number of patients who otherwise would have been excluded from the majority of programmes, namely the diabetic, elderly, and those who suffer from other medical complications. The method is ideal for use at home because unlike haemodialysis where a whole room is required for the machine, here no apparatus is needed other than the sterilized fluid and connecting tubes. Ideally there should be the integration of dialysis and transplant facilities in the one centre.

The success of renal transplantation is now indisputable, and it is as long ago as 1967 that the Medical Research Council first advised the Department of Health that the transplantation of kidneys had passed beyond the stage of pure research. The present demand for the operation is constantly in excess of supply. In February 1972, the Department of Health and Social Security set up a national organ matching service at Southmead Hospital, Bristol. The names, blood types and histo-compatibility classifications of patients waiting for kidney transplants are kept on a computer and, when donor kidneys become available, the most suitable is selected. Bristol is linked to Euro-Transplant at Leiden in Holland, which keeps a similar computerized list effecting a kidney exchange system throughout Europe.

Professor Roy Calne informed me that

'apart from living familial donation, matching for kidneys seems now to be less and less important, and cyclosporin A probably overrules what little value there is in matching. I think the concept that matching was of central importance in kidney grafting is now outdated.'

A new tissue type, the 'D system', has now been discovered, and this seems to play a more important part in whether the graft will survive. Matching of the donor kidney with the recipient for the D tissue type should produce even better results in the future.

Such is the increasing success of the operation that patient mortality at five years has fallen from close to fifty per cent to approximately ten per cent. A recent combination of improved histo-compatibility matching (DRW) and effective alternative immuno-suppression therapy (cyclosporin A) has greatly improved survival rates. It is clear that cyclosporin A represents a major advance in clinical immuno-suppression. Formerly, some fifty per cent of kidney transplants failed within the first year and patients had to be referred back to haemodialysis. With the introduction of this drug eighty per cent of patients who have had a kidney transplant now survive the critical first year.[13] This new drug has also permitted the transplant of the heart and both lungs for the first time (see p.74). The improvement which the new immunizing drug has made was made plain by Mr Terence English:

'On the whole, up until about a year or so ago, the improvement was on account of knowing more about how to use the drugs that were already available, but a couple of years ago Cyclosporin A was introduced. We started using it at Papworth in March 1982 and there are undoubted improvements. In particular both early rejection and bacterial infection have been less.'

There was a total of 1,160 cadaver kidney transplants performed in the UK and Eire during the year 1983, and the majority of patients were able to return to their full-time occupations and the support of their families. More kidney transplants are carried out in Britain per head of the population than in other large European countries, and the survival of those who have had a kidney transplant is now better than those who only have dialysis. Unfortunately in the months following the 1980 BBC Panorama programme (see p.91) the number of transplant operations fell considerably in the UK, but the number of donors has now been restored to almost the level prior to the televised programme. The waiting list for the operation has risen to 2,729 (February 1984), one third more than 1981, and the UK Transplant Service reported to the Department of Health that the number of potential kidney recipients in Britain is now more than 5,000. Yet the present supply of kidneys for transplantation is approximately a half of those required annually. In 1981 170 patients died whilst awaiting a renal transplant. Commenting on the shortage crisis, Professor Roy Calne (1982) described what is involved. 'The current annual number of operations needs to be doubled to treat the new patients and begin to reduce the backlog. There could be more than enough cadaver donors to supply all the transplantation needs. In theory, 8,000 kidneys could come from the 4,000 patients with brain death each year. In practice, some of these patients would not be suitable donors owing to the circumstances of death and the associated injuries.'[14] Many renal transplant surgeons particularly regret this acute shortage of donors because a transplant costs £6,000 plus approximately £2,000 on rehabilitation, against £55,000 for renal dialysis over five years. Also, with improved techniques transplant operations are much safer.

In the present shortage, what are some of the guidelines used for selection of patients awaiting transplant surgery? One transplant surgeon pointed out that age is a very important factor. 'Obviously, patients who are fit and will contribute back to society are extremely eligible. Apart from that, anyone who is medically fit seems to be listed. Patients who will not receive transplants are the extremely old, and those with complicating medical conditions or malignancies.' Professor Peter Morris explained:

> 'The guidelines vary obviously for the organs to be transplanted and are quite complex in the case of liver and heart recipients, but in kidney transplantation most units

would consider as acceptable all patients from the age of ten up to fifty-five, with exception being made below and above these figures by certain units. The only exclusions within this age group would be patients with severe vascular disease of the heart.'

Dr Victor Parsons described the procedure adopted in his own unit at Dulwich:

'Most of our patients are offered transplantation because it offers the best quality of life, and we would offer it to anyone irrespective of their age, sex, marital status. We don't transplant all diabetics, for instance, because some of them have advanced heart disease, and others have complications where we know transplantation won't make life very much easier for them. On the whole I think that most people who come to the end of their renal function should be offered transplantation, but a few, of course, will opt for dialysis and a few are quite untransplantable for various technical reasons.'

Kidney Donors

There are three main sources of kidney supply:

(1) *Living related donors:* The first renal transplant between a living donor and a recipient was performed in Boston 1954 (see p.47) and this was between identical twins. This is the ideal situation, for there can be no rejection. The chances of a patient having an identical twin, however, are only about 1 in 300, and even when this occurs both of the twins may be suffering from the same disease. It is understandable that a parent, brother or sister would be ready to give a kidney to their children or sibling, yet there are often ethical dilemmas arising, for when one operates on a perfectly normal healthy individual without any direct physical benefit to this patient, then small risks become more important, for it cannot be foreseen with any certainty what future problems the related donor might have. The assessment of the motivation of the donor must also be examined, and care must be taken that subtle pressures have not been forced upon him or her by

members of a closely knit family. Again a clear explanation of the risks involved should be given.

Results from living related donors are good, particularly for children who need a renal transplant (eighty to one hundred per cent in UK). There must of course be genetic similarity between the parents and the child. Normally they are out of hospital within a month with a good functioning kidney and able to return to a normal active life. Slapak (1981) records that in over 2,000 living, related kidney donations the documented mortality is less than 0.1 per cent. The long-term risk has been estimated by actual statistics as approximately that of driving a car sixteen miles every working day.[15]

(2) *Living unrelated donors:* There may be a well-meaning individual who is not related to the potential recipient and who is eager to help. The results in these instances are not good and present further ethical problems. Such a source of donor is rarely used in the UK as results are variable, and no better than with cadaveric donors. In the Federal Republic of Germany and Switzerland live donor transplantation is not undertaken as it is considered unethical. In the UK 117 live donor transplants were undertaken in 1980.[16]

Professor Roy Calne (1975) recommends that the donor be told that the operation is painful and not devoid of risk, and that should he injure his remaining kidney subsequently, there would be no reserve of renal function. Also, the chances of the graft being successful in the recipient should be fully explained. It is important too that the doctor should not put pressure on unwilling relatives to donate. Repeated contact with the family is desirable, so that the doctor can eliminate with some degree of confidence intra-familial pressures on an unwilling donor. If there is any doubt he feels it is best to avoid living donors.[17]

Although the younger the donor is the better are the chances of success, the BMA *Handbook of Medical Ethics* (1981) firmly and emphatically states that 'there are no circumstances in which a child can be considered a suitable donor of non-regenerative tissue. There is no legal certainty about a parent's right to give consent on behalf of the child, but if this exists that right cannot extend to any procedure which is not

in the child's best interests' (p. 36). In the majority of instances it is now only brain dead patients on ventilators who are
considered as potential donors.

(3) *Cadaveric donors:* In most countries between seventy and
ninety per cent of all renal transplants are from cadaveric
donors, and in Great Britain alone over ninety per cent of
kidneys used are from this source. The majority of kidneys
would have been obtained from persons with irreversible
brain damage, caused in the main by road accidents (sixty-
five per cent). Intracerebral catastrophes due to intracranial
haemorrhage form a further twenty-six per cent of cadaveric
donors, and the third most common group includes primary
brain tumours after unsuccessful surgical intervention. The
donor should preferably be a young person, with no history of
hypertension, malignant disease or infection. Age is important
as the older the kidney the less well it subsequently works.
The kidney has to be removed within ninety minutes of the
circulation ceasing.

Cardiac Transplantation

At present heart transplantation seems to be becoming less
and less an experimental procedure and more a routine clinical treatment. Of those who have undergone the operation
two out of three survive at least a year, and the best teams in
the United States have survival rates of more than five years
for one in two patients and several over ten years. At an
International Meeting of the Transplant Society at Brighton
(August 1982), significant improvements in the long-term
survival rate of heart and liver transplant patients were
reported. Surgical methods, tissue typing and post-operative
nursing have all contributed to this advance. Leading surgeons both in the UK and the USA attributed much of the
higher success rate to the new drug cyclosporin A in helping to
combat rejection (see p.73). One group (Professor Norman
Shumway, Stanford, USA) which was the first to use the drug
for heart transplant reported that the one year survival rate
had risen from two in three to four in five.

Results in some of the US centres confirm that human heart
transplantation may now be considered therapeutic rather
than experimental, for results are comparable to those for

renal transplantation in units at Oxford, Cambridge, and Minneapolis, USA. Ninety per cent of surviving cardiac recipients in the Stanford (USA) programme have returned to full activity and the majority have resumed active employment.[18]

French heart transplant patient Emmanuel Vitra celebrated the fifteenth anniversary of his operation in December 1983. The longest surviving British heart transplant patient, Mr Keith Castle, received his new heart at Papworth Hospital in August 1979. Since cardiac transplantations commenced at Harefield and Papworth Hospitals in that year (1979), almost two hundred patients have received a cardiac transplant. This number includes the 'piggy-back' operations performed by Mr Magdi Yacoub's team at Harefield Hospital, in which a donor heart is linked in parallel with a failing heart.

The prospects for survival for twelve months are now better than eight in ten. Once past this initial stage the five year survival rate is expected to be ninety per cent. Up to 1982 more than 750 cardiac transplantations had been performed in 74 countries.

The latest development has been the insertion of a plastic heart worked by compressed air. A team of doctors in Salt Lake City made medical history on 2 December, 1982, when they gave Dr Barney Clark, a 61-year-old dentist from Seattle, a polyurethane and aluminium heart. The artificial heart weighed 10 ounces, and was lined with a soft dacron velvet mesh which minimized the damage to red blood cells. It consisted of two similarly constructed halves; one half pumps blood to the lungs, the other pumps blood round the body just as a natural heart functions. The patient survived a few months (112 days).

The best donors, as with renal transplants, are young people who have suffered irreversible brain damage as a result of cerebral trauma or haemorrhage. Ideally the heart should be removed while it is still beating from a patient with brain death. While the one team removes the donor heart the second team puts the recipient on total cardiac by-pass with the heart-lung machine and excises the recipient's heart. The heart must be removed within fifteen minutes of the circulation ceasing.

At Papworth Hospital, Cambridge, Mr Terence English

outlined some of his criteria for the selection of patients for heart transplantation. They have at Papworth

> 'defined criteria which exclude both the young, below the age of fifteen, and the older, above the age of fifty. It was a difficult decision and an entirely arbitrary one, and it was taken by me because I knew that our resources were restricted, not only in terms of hearts but also in terms of money. The Stanford programme had shown that people above the age of fifty did not tolerate the procedure particularly well, and certainly not as well as the younger patients. For the younger range I did not want to offer anything that was as unpredictable as a heart transplant to a child who could not understand the implications of what was being offered, and for whom the decision would therefore have to be taken by the parents.'

Mr English then went on to describe the programme of assessment which takes place prior to the operation itself. It was a fascinating account:

> 'All the family is concerned in this programme of assessment', he explained. 'They are told about the risks and the imponderables — the very fact that we cannot predict a good result; that probably a quarter will die in the first year after a heart transplant, and that I can't tell Mr X whether he will be in that group or not. I also point out that because of the shortage of donor hearts we only transplant just over half of those whom we accept. We try and make their period of assessment a process of education. They have the opportunity to talk to other patients who have had the operation, social workers, psychiatrists, and at the end of the four to five days I generally give them our conclusion. I don't tend to give them strong advice but either offer to accept them on the programe or not. It has to be that way for the first decision has to be theirs, and they can only make up their minds if they are informed. For this reason we spend a lot of time discussing all aspects of the procedure with them. If they ask me specifically how long they are likely to live if they did not have a transplant then I try to give them

an answer. Previously doctors looking after them may have tried to dodge that question but usually the patients know they are seriously ill and deteriorating, and I think it can be a great relief for them to talk about their condition and their future in a frank and open way. There is also the element of hope that transplantation offers, and I believe this has sustained many who unfortunately died before they could be transplanted. Very often it is the wives who need more counselling than the patients.'

In the further development of cardiac transplantation two major constraints appear to be: (1) the limited supply of suitable donor organs, and (2) the financial cost of establishing and maintaining clinical programmes.

(1) In practice, as English and Cory-Pearce (1981) explain, the supply of organs is determined to a large extent by medical and public attitudes towards central issues such as the diagnosis of brain death and the appropriateness or otherwise of organ transplantation. The majority of their donor hearts during the past two and a half years have resulted from relatives spontaneously offering heart donation after having been asked for kidney donation, rather than from doctors specifically asking for heart donation. This emphasizes how dependent cardiac transplantation is on favourable public attitudes.[19]

(2) A strong case is made for putting financial resources into preventive cardiological medicine so reducing the 150,000 deaths a year from coronary heart disease. A heart transplant costs approximately twice as much as a kidney recipient, and twenty-five times the cost of a hip replacement operation. It is argued that control of smoking, obesity and hypertension would save many more lives than cardiac transplantation could ever hope to save. The Office of Health Economies (a research body formed by the pharmaceutical industry) has estimated that at least 2,000 lives could be saved each year by screening for and treating raised blood pressure.[20] Are then such transplant operations justifiable within the present limitations of current financial resources and manpower? Mr

P. J. Wilson gave an unreserved 'yes' to kidney transplantation but

> 'in relation to heart, heart-lung, liver, pancreas transplants we must admit some serious reservations', he confessed. 'It is likely that time and experience will lessen these reservations. Transplants will *always* be costly. However, *real* doctors have to concern themselves with their *real* individual patients and not with abstract considerations of some general good. This, of course, is the essential doctor's dilemma, isn't it?'

Somewhat similar views were expressed by Professor Peter Morris:

> 'Kidney transplants are fully justifiable as they provide the probability of restoring patients in the productive phase of their lives to a state where they can become a full and productive member of society. The cheapest outcome in a time of limited resources is of course failure to provide treatment of any sort, with death of the patient. However, if one does have to provide dialysis then transplantation of a kidney becomes a much cheaper solution as well as providing a much higher proportion of patients fully rehabilitated.'

The costs of liver and heart transplants

> 'are rather more and in terms of the results less justified at the present time. However, if such procedures are not done in a limited number of centres then the opportunity to develop these procedures at a time when some of the major immunological problems have been solved will be limited.'

According to Mr Michael Bewick dialysis is not an economical prospect:

> 'It does cost £10,000 a year to keep a patient going on a machine and that is expensive, and very often the patient is not back at work, and therefore not back in the economy — a drain on the economy of the country. Therefore transplantation — apart from the medical expediency, its economic expediency is overwhelming.'

Dr Victor Parsons and his hospital had looked at the costing of transplantation in detail:

> 'It works out about £5/6,000 per year for a whole year and of course the next year, if it's successful, is much less; its something in the order of £1,500 per year from then on. When we look at other areas of medicine, which is the only real comparison we can make with the value of what we do medically, then we can say that we certainly are offering a much cheaper form of treatment than any other long-term disabled patient. To keep a heavily disabled person in hospital is in the order of £20,000 per year and no one suggests that they shouldn't be kept alive or looked after well.'

As far as the social worth is concerned, Dr Parsons continued:

> 'Compared to what is done in society to prevent people dying, it is even cheaper. You will spend very much more money on a motorway to make it safe, or on a block of flats so that it doesn't collapse, or various other measures. The preventative things that people are quite willing to pay for in society as a whole are far more expensive than what we are doing. So, if society can afford that, we feel we can justifiably ask for £5,000 per year for our transplant patients.'

The proponents of cardiac transplantation point out that the cost of such operations and subsequent treatment has to be weighed against that of keeping a person invalided. They state that most patients are family men in their forties to mid-fifties, so that there is an economic return as well as a relief of human suffering in restoring a patient to active life. It is interesting to note that over the last two years the cost of heart transplants has halved. Shorter stays in hospital after surgery have contributed to a reduction in the cost of each operation from between £17,000 and £20,000 in 1982 to £10,000 in 1984. These figures are inclusive of the cost of the initial assessment, the operation and care over the subsequent twelve months. Many patients who undergo cardiac transplant surgery are now able to leave hospital after a stay of four to six weeks instead of remaining in hospital, as previously, for three to six months.

When I enquired about the possibilities in the future of artificial hearts being inserted, Mr Terence English thought they were still quite a long way off and associated with enormous development costs:

> 'They have the money to spend on this in the USA. I think eventually we shall reach the stage of artificial hearts, but they will be unlikely to be viable within the next ten years, so I think there is quite an important immediate future for human heart transplantation.'

Liver Transplantation

Liver transplantations have various technical problems which make it among the most difficult of transplant operations with which to succeed. The first liver transplant took place in 1963 at Denver, USA. Starzl has performed about 370 of the estimated 600 liver transplants that have been undertaken throughout the world. In 1968 liver transplants were commenced in the Cambridge/King's College Hospital series and their number of cases has now reached well over 100. The donor criteria are identical to those for renal transplantation, i.e. complete and irreversible cerebral death requiring maintenance on a ventilator. The liver must be removed within fifteen minutes of the circulation ceasing.

Unlike the unsuccessful renal recipient who can be put back on haemodialysis and undergo further transplants when necessary, there is no such rescue or safety net for the unsuccessful liver transplant patient. With the introduction of the use of cyclosporin A the one-year rates of graft and patient survival have more than doubled and are now sixty-five to seventy per cent. Previously the survival rate resulted in only thirty per cent after the first year. Twenty out of 108 liver recipients are alive, six are surviving more than five years after surgery; the longest survivor in the UK is nearly eight years. Many are now able to lead completely normal lives doing full-time work and are active in sport.[21] Many patients who would have died from untreatable liver disease have now been restored to normal life for several years, and the operation is probably less costly than prolonged care of a patient dying of liver disease in hospital. The longest survivor after orthotopic liver allografting is a patient of Professor Thomas Starzl

(Denver, USA), well more than fourteen years after the operation. One patient at Denver has given birth to two normal children after transplantation. As a number of patients accepted for transplantation die while awaiting the operation, and more donor organs are needed, centres in Groningen, Cambridge, and Denver have developed a liver-sharing scheme.

Heart-Lung and Pancreas Transplantations

Such operations have improved over the past five years but the technical problems of such transplantations still remain difficult. The heart-lung procedure has been perfected by the team of Professor Norman Shumway at Stanford University, California, where the first heart-lung transplant was done in March 1981. Sixteen patients have been given new organs. Five have died but all the others have returned to normal life. Irrespective of any conceivable advance in artificial organs, Professor Shumway sees heart-lung transplantation as here to stay.[22] The results of the combined operation are far better than those attempted for just lung transplantation. The longest survivor is alive two and a half years after the operation. On 6 December 1983 the first heart-lung transplant in the UK was carried out at Harefield Hospital. Heart-lung transplants are not seen as a treatment suitable for a large number of people. Only ten to twelve patients a year in Britain are likely to undergo such surgery if the procedure becomes established. Pancreas grafting is still experimental, but results are encouraging

> 'We don't really know the result', Professor Roy Calne stated, 'whether this is going to be a valuable tool. Of course, if it is shown to be of great benefit to diabetics then pancreas grafting could be one of the most important developments in the future.'

Conclusions

Are transplant patients (liver, heart) being given a meaningful level of life, or a rather prolonged state of suffering and need? All the physicians and surgeons with whom I discussed this question were optimistic. I was reassured by Professor Peter Morris:

'A successful renal transplant provides the recipient with virtually a normal quality of life. Some eighty per cent of recipients of successful kidney transplants are fully rehabilitated. However, liver and heart recipients at this point in time have a rather lower success rate and a less satisfactory quality of life. Nevertheless, this situation is altering for the better as time goes on.'

Another transplant surgeon gave a similar optimistic testimony: 'Patients are being given an extremely meaningful level of life. They are certainly not being kept in a prolonged state of suffering and need.' Making reference to kidney transplantation in particular, he continued: 'Many patients desire transplant but cannot receive it, and therefore tolerate dialysis as a way of existence. What is more important is that patients who could benefit from dialysis and transplantation may not be receiving this therapy because there are not enough facilities to treat them.'

A more cautious note came from Mr P. J. Wilson:

'In kidney transplants, *usually* the former applies. In liver and heart transplants, *sometimes* the former applies. But no transplant recipient can ever escape from close medical supervision. However worthwhile their lives, they live on borrowed time.'

If vital organ transplantations are justified in terms of finance, are they justified in terms of results produced? The consultants to whom I spoke had no reservations at all.

'I wish you could see my kidney transplant out-patients' clinic!' exclaimed Dr Mary McGeown from Belfast.

Results certainly seem most encouraging. 'The results have got better over the last ten years. Certainly in the last two years, results have improved due to a few advances, i.e. cyclosporin A and blood transfusion,' one of the surgeons remarked. 'One cannot look down upon the transplant success results of eighty to ninety per cent.'

Dr Victor Parsons was quite happy that things are improving, techniques are getting better, and there are new drugs:

'We feel it is giving a good quality of life to a proportion of patients which is well justified.'

Mr Terence English gave me his survival figures for heart transplantation:

> 'The longest survivor we have at present is Mr Keith Castle who is now just over four years since his transplant, and three of my first six patients are still alive. At present (October 1983) there are fifty-eight patients that have been transplanted of whom thirty-five are alive at present. Most of the deaths occur early, that is, in the first three to six months. I think our one year survival rate to date is about sixty per cent. After that the outlook improves and there's much less likelihood of patients dying from rejection during the next five years or so. The best results have come from Professor Shumway's group at Stanford, USA, where the one year survival is now approximately seventy-five per cent.'

Mr X had recently undergone cardiac transplantation and I discussed with him his feelings about the operation in his room on the intensive care unit:

> 'All I can say to you', remarked Mr X, 'is that I feel as if something quite miraculous has happened to me and really that I've been given a new life. The disease from which I was suffering first struck me down about two and a half years ago. Latterly I was taking thousands of tablets a year. I had to stop work — I could not work — and I gradually became chairbound, but never completely chairbound, thank God. I always managed to get on my feet every day, but I had long spells in hospital. When I was home I did not get a complete night's sleep for over three to four months, and there were times when I was coughing continuously day and night. So that was the state I was in . . . eventually I was referred to this hospital for consideration for transplantation. When the idea of transplantation was suggested to me my reaction at that time was that I was not opposed to the idea of transplantation on any moral or ethical grounds, because I consider that it is a perfectly justified surgical procedure if we are to progress in medicine.'

Mr X described his visit to the hospital for 'assessment'.

'Every question I asked was answered, no matter how silly it appeared, and we were positively encouraged to ask these questions. Items which had been worrying me didn't worry me any longer, I think because they had been explained to me. I eventually arrived 6.20 pm — I was prepared for the operation and certainly by 4 o'clock the next morning I had my new heart in. Now to this date I do not know anything about the donor side, but I just thank whoever gave their heart to me.'

He went on to speak of his post-operative period:

'The progress in my own case has been very, very rapid; in fact, twelve days exactly to the minute almost, I was told that my barrier nursing could come off, and twelve days after I walked into this hospital I walked through the door of my temporary bubble. I am now sitting here some twenty days on from admission. When we met I had just come back from a good two mile walk around the grounds of this hospital without any ill effects whatsoever — a hard walk, I wasn't ambling, I was striding — so far, please God, everything is rock steady?'

I asked Mr X what his feelings were now the operation was over:

'To me it must be some sort of miracle. Now I'm not and never have been an adherent of organized religion — I suppose I'm the fairly typical man who has an early religious background and has a feeling — yes, there is 'something'! But as a result of this I think that one comes to accept the existence of some Power. How many times have we all said: "If only I could live my life again". Now some of us have been given this opportunity . . . What would you prefer, to sit in that chair for two years like a cabbage or have six months, one year, or more of active vigorous life. What would your choice be?'

On the question of after-care Mr X commented:

'One still has to come back here regularly for tests which go on, and really for the rest of one's life one is involved in this programme. After all, we are given an awful lot

and we have to return this in a practical way of helping
with the research programme. As far as any moral or
ethical aspects are concerned each person will have his
own belief on this. My own belief is that we were not
given this facility by God in order to waste it, but to use
it.'

How did Mr X look to the future?

'I feel I'm only here to give now, not to take. What I
mean to say is, I've been given so much that I must give
some back, and in whatever way I can do this I will —
that will be my future.'[23]

There seem no particular ethical problems concerned with
the transplantation of the above organs once (1) the concept of
brain death has been accepted (see Chapter 3), (2) there is a
real probability of benefit to the recipient, (3) there is full trust
and confidence in the medical profession.

The reservation of some Roman Catholic moralists towards
the use of live donors on the 'principle of totality', which
distinguishes between a justifiable and unjustifiable
'mutation' or invasion of a person's bodily integrity, is coun-
terbalanced by the attitude of much contemporary Roman
Catholic thought, which sees organ donation from a living
donor as a humane and charitable contribution to another
fellow human being who is less fortunate than oneself. Such a
self-sacrifice on behalf of another is seen as both legitimate
and laudable.[24]

The strongest argument used to justify human transplantation is that based on christian charity. Man does not have
full dominion over his life, and the donation of an organ is an
expression of that self-sacrificing love which a Christian
should have for his neighbour.

It is interesting to note that the Code of Practice, *Cadaveric
Organs for Transplantation* (1983), states:- 'As far as is known no
major religious grouping in the UK objects outright to the
principle of organ donation and transplantation, although
there are some who feel it is only permissible if the donor
himself requested it before he died. These include in particu-

lar, Orthodox Jews, Muslims, Hindus and Christian Scientists. The Jehovah's Witnesses have religious objection to blood transfusions, but feel that donating or receiving organs is a matter for each Jehovah's Witness to decide for himself.' Jewish Law insists that no vital organ be removed from a donor until death is definitely established by the actual cessation of all essential life functions, including particularly respiration and pulsation, and not merely by what is termed 'clinical death', such as irreversible brain damage.[25]

The above Report also emphasizes how very important is the approach to relatives, which should be made with proper sensitivity and feeling for the relatives' distress. It suggests that the persons best qualified to approach the family apart from a member of the transplant team ought to be a senior nurse (e.g. ward sister), a chaplain or the family doctor (p. 8).

Not only can such transplantations bring much benefit to the recipients themselves but also they can often bring a certain degree of satisfaction and emotional benefit to sorrowing relatives. At the Radcliffe Infirmary, Oxford, it has been the practice to write and thank the donor's family and relatives and inform them of the result of the transplantation. A reply such as the following shows what support a bereaved family can derive from an organ(s) being donated on behalf of another. 'My wife, son and I were given considerable pleasure at this bleak time by your kind letter. We hope the recipient of our daughter's kidney continues to make good progress and we are proud that we could help someone whose recovery was a practical proposition. Perhaps you would kindly tell the recipient that the parents of the donor wish her well and hope she has a happy, healthy life as a result of your surgery. Thanking you for writing to us . . .'.[26]

There is need for great respect and care as to how organs for transplantation are procured, with full respect to the dignity of man and proper reverence for the human body made in the image of God. Every consideration must also be given to see that by concentrating both skilled manpower and extra finance on such operations with comparatively few patients, the many in need of other surgical and medical treatments do not suffer loss or deprivation.

The author wishes to acknowledge his gratitude to Roy Calne, Professor of Surgery, University of Cambridge, for commenting upon and reading through the original draft of this chapter for medical accuracy.

3
Brain Death

Death has always been determined by the absence of function — the cessation of spontaneous ventilation (breathing) and the stoppage of the heartbeat. This concept still applies in the majority of instances. It was clear that when the respiration and heart stopped the brain would die in a few minutes, so the obvious criterion of no heartbeat being synonymous with death was sufficiently accurate. The heart was considered to be the central and most important organ of the body and its failure to function was the mark of death. Illustrations of Victorian deathbed scenes often depicted a feather or a mirror being held close to the dying person's mouth or nostrils to ascertain whether breathing had actually stopped or not. Shakespeare in *King Lear* describes such a procedure.

'I know when one is dead and when one lives,
She's dead as earth, Lend me a looking glass,
If that her breath will mist or stain the stone,
Why, then she lives.'

Under most circumstances the cessation of spontaneous respiration and heartbeat are still perfectly adequate and standard signs of death, but the patients under discussion are those who have sustained acute, massive, irreparable brain damage which has put them into irreversible coma. Their respiration has stopped due to irrecoverable brain damage but their circulation is still intact because they are being maintained on artificial ventilation.

What precisely does it mean to say the brain is dead? What part of the brain? Mr Peter Wilson gave a full and graphic definition:

'Brain death means total and irrevocable cessation of all the neurological functions that subserve independent breathing, sensation, volition, reflex action, thought, memory, personality, consciousness, bodily homoeostasis. The *entire* brain may be so affected but specifically it is the *brain stem* that we consider and test in arriving at the diagnosis. Needless to say, there must in all cases be absolute objective demonstration of a clinical and investigative context compatible with irrevocability, e.g. massive brain injury or haemorrhage. Brain death *can* be obvious within only a few moments: usually we re-test at intervals for up to several days.'

Professor J. K. Mason went on to emphasize how important it is to speak of brain stem death rather than brain death, for

'apart from the fact that the rest of the brain will almost certainly be dead if the part most resistant to anoxia — the brain stem — is dead, the term removes any semantic difficulty. The brain stem is responsible for the maintenance of the vital cardio-respiratory functions. If the brain stem is dead the body is unable to sustain a separate existence and is, therefore, dead. It follows that to continue ventilation in the presence of brain stem death is merely to ventilate a corpse.'

At BMA House I further discussed the function of the brain stem with Professor Bryan Jennett as we talked together about various aspects of brain death:

'The brain stem sends impulses in two directions, downwards to the breathing, which is why the breathing stops when the brain is dead; and upwards to activate the cortex. So even if the cortex, the grey matter, is intact and quite healthy, if you chop off the brain stem it switches off the cortex.'

It is reported that there are about four thousand brain deaths a year in British hospitals, which is under one per cent of all deaths. Half the cases of such brain deaths occur as a result of recent head injury, while spontaneous intracranial haemorrhage accounts for about another third.[1]

Need to update death
With the introduction of modern resuscitative and supportive measures (the mechanical lung ventilator, haemodialysis, intensive care units, organ transplantation and supportive

therapies in the 1950s), the traditional definition of death (i.e. cessation of breathing and heartbeat) is no longer valid, for these modern technological procedures can now restore 'life' as conceived by the traditional standards of persistent (albeit artificial) respiration and continuing natural heartbeat. When a patient has to receive such artificial life support (the ventilator) these various procedures make the application of the traditional simple criteria difficult, for by use of mechanical ventilation the heart and the lungs are able to function but the brain remains in a non-functional state.

Is that individual patient alive, we may well ask, for although he has a heart that beats he is unable to breathe naturally? If patients in this condition were to be left in intensive care units indefinitely, however, not only would such hospital units soon be overtaxed and the medical and nursing staff demoralised, but also it would be extremely grievous for next of kin to see their loved ones being mechanically sustained with no chance of recovery to normal life. A logical development therefore was that a new concept of death was introduced — brain death, based upon the demonstration of a non-functioning brain. It should be made clear, however, that not all patients with brain damage who are on ventilators have brain death; even of those with extensive and irrecoverable brain damage only some are brain dead.[2]

It is now officially accepted that when the brain has irreversibly ceased to function, for example, on account of overwhelming head injury, then the person is dead in spite of the fact that respiration (and consequently the circulation) are artificially maintained. 'Irreversibility' is the key word. This is further clarified by the statement (section 4) in the memorandum of the Conference of Medical Royal Colleges and their Faculties in the UK (see p.96): 'It is now universally accepted, by the lay public as well as by the medical profession, that it is not possible to equate death itself with cessation of heartbeat. Quite apart from the elective cardiac arrest of open heart surgery, spontaneous cardiac arrest followed by a successful resuscitation is today a commonplace and although the more sensational accounts of occurrences of this kind still refer to the patient as being "dead" until restoration of the heartbeat, the use of the quote marks usually demonstrates that this word is not to be taken literally, for to most people the one aspect of death that is beyond debate is its irreversibility.'

So deeply rooted is the traditional cessation of cardiac activity that it is extremely difficult for a lay person, brought up to believe that heart and respiratory functions are signs of life and their non-functioning indicates death, to acknowledge that a diagnosis of death can now be confirmed in patients whose hearts are still beating. There is too the additional difficulty of differentiating the process of dying from the fact of death. The importance traditionally accorded to a person's beating heart in distinguishing the living from the dead is further challenged when a 'dead' person's heart can now beat in the chest of a 'living' person, whose own heart has not merely stopped but has been removed from his or her body. Old concepts and traditions die hard and the subject of death is still highly emotive. It has to be borne in mind that from a biological standpoint there can be no such thing as 'the precise moment of death', for death is a process rather than an event.

In the past, and to a certain extent in the present, there seems to lurk in the minds of a number of people an innate fear of being buried alive.[3] In the last century elaborate precautions were often devised; coffins were constructed with a bell-rope dangling next to the corpse's head and mortuaries were designed to allow continuous surveillance of bodies for two or three days prior to burial. The invention of the stethoscope in the mid-nineteenth century did much to allay such public fears of premature burial for it enabled the physician to detect heartbeat with a high degree of sensitivity.

With the advent of organ transplantation over the past decades and as staff of intensive care units became more and more skilled in maintaining deeply unconscious patients alive for days and sometimes for weeks, these trepidations were replaced somewhat by the thought that organs might be removed for transplant operations while life was still extant. One comparatively recent survey[4] showed that one reason why certain people did not carry a kidney donor card was the fear that their organs might be taken from their bodies before they were actually dead. Many people questioned — would surgeons become so over-zealous that death might be prematurely announced? Such fears were further accentuated by rather florid accounts in national newspapers of patients moving as incisions were made in operating theatres to remove organs! Headlines referred to some members of surgical transplantation teams as 'vultures', searching for all possible human organs which could be transplanted into suitable donors! Many of the general public understandably associated brain death with organ transplantation operations, and some still seem rather suspicious about the accuracy of the diagnosis of brain death for this very reason. (see p.86) But organ transplantation should be seen as an entirely different issue from that of brain death, and the loyalties of individual doctors quite undivided. Indeed in the majority of brain death patients the question of organ transplantation does not even arise. Only one brain dead patient out of every four or five becomes a donor, even in those units which are committed to securing organs.[5] The conclusion that brain death has occurred is reached entirely independently of any transplant considerations. Very wisely the Royal Colleges' criteria do not make mention of transplantation.

When a diagnosis of brain death has been confirmed, however, the provision of organs can be considered and discussed discreetly with the patient's next of kin, for organs removed from brain dead patients have a much better opportunity of providing successful function than organs removed after primary circulatory arrest.

The diagnosis of brain death therefore became even more pertinent as transplant surgery developed and donor organs were required as early as possible (after a patient has been two or three days on a ventilator, infection, low blood pressure etc. make organs unsuitable for transplantation). As the majority of transplant surgeons are unwilling to use organs, particularly kidneys, from other than beating heart cadavers, the pronouncement of death must be on the basis of brain death. The need for a 'definition' of brain death was also required for the relief of the next of kin and relatives of patients who were on ventilators in indefinitely prolonged coma. In the words of Dr Christopher Pallis (1983), 'they become emotional hostages to uncomprehending machines', and he gives four sound reasons why it is bad to 'ventilate a corpse'.[6] There is the obvious distress to relatives; it is bad for morale of nursing staff; limited facilities are being denied to those who might benefit from them; and there is the cost-effectiveness equation. On all these counts it seemed only logical to introduce a new concept of death based upon the demonstration of a permanently non-functioning brain.

Some Misconceptions

(1) Mistaken Diagnosis: Sometimes one reads in the popular press of instances of patients recovering who have supposedly been considered 'brain dead', and such reports in turn have led to allegations that brain death has been mistakenly diagnosed. Let it be said that not one of these instances has been corroborated. Reflex limb movements can occur in response to certain stimuli, for the spinal cord function sometimes persists after brain death. Such patients have some appearance of life, a moving chest, pulsing blood vessels and bodily warmth, all of which can understandably confuse the uninitiated into believing that recovery from brain death is possible and may prompt them to ask, or to wonder, might there not therefore be some flicker of awareness remaining inside the unconscious patient's brain?

(2) Drug Intoxication: Profound yet irreversible changes in brain stem function may also be caused by drug intoxication, hypothermia and metabolic or endocrine disturbances, and these can in turn produce states akin to brain death. Doctors therefore must always check for drugs before testing for brain stem death, for in the presence of certain drugs brain death should not be considered (see UK Code p. 100). Hypothermia and the possible use of depressant drugs must always be most vigorously excluded before any diagnosis of brain death be confirmed. The Brodick Committee on Death Certification (1974) further clarifies the issue: 'Two of the three recently reported cases of patients recovering after once having been given up for dead have concerned persons, who, before their bodies were examined by doctors, had taken large quantities of tablets containing barbiturates'. It further explains that such extreme coma induced by barbiturates 'could be mis-

taken for death because it appears to eliminate breathing and heart beat, chills the body and produces deep unconsciousness with weak or totally non-existent reflexes'.[7]

I asked a number of doctors how long a patient could remain in a state of drug-induced coma? How soon after admission to hospital can it be safely stated that the patient's condition is *not* due to drugs? How available are toxicological facilities?

> 'If there is any suspicion at all of a coma having been induced by drugs', explained Dr Mary McGeown, 'at least 48 hours are allowed to elapse before considering doing the tests for brain death. In such cases at least a further 24 hours would be allowed to elapse and the tests repeated. There is no urgency to reach a diagnosis of brain death with a patient on a respirator, as such a patient would be. There is plenty of time to allow the situation to be assessed repeatedly until every one concerned is satisfied.'

Mr Maurice Slapak affirmed that

> 'drug induced comas can only be declared brain dead if, (a) the drug ingested is known, (b) its blood level is negligible for over 24 hours, (c) during that 24 hours there is no evidence of any amelioration of brain function as measured by repeated EEG as well as by clinical tests.'

On the question of the availability of toxicological facilities it seems that they are reasonably widely available on a supra-regional basis although, according to Professor Morris, 'not immediately available in most centres'. Professor Jennett assured me there were 24 hour-a-day centres but only in a small minority of instances where it becomes a major issue.

> 'Time is the big factor', he stated. 'If there's any suspicion of drugs, wait 24 hours, 48 hours, wait 72 hours if there is any doubt. But in most cases that doubt doesn't exist and you do not have to do a toxicological test on every case.'

(3) Vegetative State: A clear distinction must be drawn

between the death of the brain and a prolonged or irreversible state of coma (see Havard Ad Hoc Committee p.94). These two terms are not synonymous and describe different states. The term 'irreversible coma' should not be used when the vegetative state is being described. Although the condition may be irreversible the patient in the vegetative state is *not* comatose, because there are periods when he/she is awake (eyes open and moving) — although never aware. Karen Quinlan, for example, is in a vegetative state.[8] Cerebral death denotes total lack of function of the brain, so that both volitional reflex evidence of responsivity are lacking. It involves complete unresponsiveness to stimuli above the spinal cord, lack of respiratory effort and absence of brain stem reflexes. In the 'vegetative state', on the other hand, all functions attributed to the cerebrum are lost but certain vital functions such as respiration, temperature and blood pressure regulation may be retained, together with spinal reflexes. Professor Bryan Jennett (1972), who with Fred Plum first coined the phrase 'persistent vegetative state'[9] to describe this condition, states that 'the patient can . . . breathe and swallow (although often requiring tube feeding) but he has no psychological meaningful responses to the environment. No words are uttered, but there are periods of wakefulness when the eyes open, and they may follow moving objects reflexly . . . such patients can survive for years, given adequate nursing support'. The condition is often referred to as 'awake but unaware'.[10]

How long such patients who are in a state of 'living death' (indeed many would go so far as to describe the vegetative state as worse than death) should be allowed to survive is an acute ethical, legal and social problem. Can 'human life' be attributed to a patient whose cerebral cortex has been completely destroyed and who survives in a state of irreversible coma? Legally such patients are alive although the quality of life is extremely limited. Gordon Dunstan makes the helpful comment that such a patient 'is not "kept alive" — he lives. And while he lives, he is entitled to elementary human care, that is, nursing care, simply to be fed, turned, kept clean. Whether an attack of pneumonia, say, should be countered with active therapy, like an antibiotic, is another question; appropriate management might rather be to let the body fight its own battle, win or lose — there is no obligation in such a case, to administer a particular therapy.'

It is a serious ethical and moral consideration for both doctors and families, whether or not such patients should be maintained by extraordinary means for indefinite periods when they will never be able to share in the interpersonal relationships which characterize a normal individual. Pope Pius XII addressing a Congress of Anaesthetists in November 1957, on 'Prolongation of Life', stated that 'human life continues for as long as its vital functions, distinguished from the simple life of the organs, manifest themselves without the help of artificial processes'. He added, 'Normally one is held to use only ordinary means — according to the circumstances of persons, places, times and cultures — that is to say, means that do not involve any grave burdens for oneself or another . . . It remains for the doctor to give a clear and precise definition of death, and the "moment of death" of a patient who passes away in the state of unconsciousness.'

The majority of doctors would probably consider it good medical practice not to intervene actively by giving antibiotics should complications develop, and would seek the consent of the family for such a policy. Yet one can well appreciate the soul searching required by the doctor who throughout his long training has been taught to do everything possible to save life. Even with the 'informed consent' of the next of kin it still remains for the physician a delicate and difficult judgement. The following extract from an annotation in *The Lancet* (1974) proffers some sound advice for the physician in the dilemma confronting him and seems to express the general attitude of the medical profession: 'When a patient who already has severe brain damage develops respiratory insufficiency or cardiorespiratory arrest, careful thought should be taken before artificial respiration is extended beyond the immediate resuscitation period. Prolongation of such a patient's life, even for twelve hours (it may often be much longer in practice) reflects no credit on his doctor, particularly if this is done only so as to postpone the decision to let events take their natural course. It would be unfortunate if the time came when no patient in hospital could decently die without the last rite of modern medicine — a statutory period on the ventilator'.[11]

When I discussed such questions with Professor Mason he affirmed that as death is an absolute

> 'therefore, often regrettably, a person in the persistent vegetative state of Jennett is not dead and must be treated as a live patient. But once the possibility of recovery has been ruled out, there is every justification for applying the ordinary/extraordinary treatment test or, as I prefer it, the productive/non-productive test. Prolonging non-sentient dying is non-productive. Such cases should be ventilated for diagnostic purposes — not for treatment — which draws attention to the important principle that the major ethical decision in brain damaged cases is *admitting* the patient to the ventilator rather than withdrawing support.'

This seems to be the opinion of the majority of doctors. Peter Wilson was also for no 'heroics':

> 'In such cases all ordinary nursing attention, including nutrition, should be given, irrespective of age. No drugs should (or need) be given. No heroic, interventionist, extraordinary, or supererogatory treatments of a medical, surgical, "scientific", or "research" description should be applied, either in cold blood or if some sudden deterioration or relapse occurs, however theoretically "treatable" such deterioration may be.'

Professor Morris confessed to it being a very difficult problem to resolve and outlined some of the reasons why:

> 'Intuitively one would feel that the patient with severe brain damage without demonstrable brain death requiring artificial means of survival should have such means withdrawn after a reasonable period of time. However, the predictability of recovery is uncertain in a very small number of cases. But even here it would seem reasonable to set a time limit on how long artificial means of support should be maintained.'

The need of a time limit was a point taken up by Mr Maurice Slapak who submitted that:

> 'a consensus agreement between relatives, doctors and some "general public opinion" representative may be a

useful way of agreeing to terminate after an appropriately adequate period of time — *months* not weeks.'

How difficult it was to reach such a decision and to take such responsibility was expressed by Dr Victor Parsons:

'You might say after a period of a few months when everything has settled down and is static — right, the time has come — but it's very, very difficult. Sometimes families get exhausted by the situation as well and you might say to them, "If a further complication occurred do you wish further measures to be taken?" and they usually say, "No". That means that if the patient does develop pneumonia or their heart stops, then nothing else would be done. The final illness should *be* the final illness!'

Professor Jennett maintained that there were a number of doctors both in USA and here who believe that

'we should try to find some means of withdrawing treatment — treatment being "feeding and watering". Such patients require to be fed, and if they weren't fed they would die. I think the reluctance to move explicitly to that is the argument of "the slippery slope" — it would be the mentally handicapped and/or the geriatric cases next. I have always reserved my position on this. It has to be treated with all the circumspection and all the reservation that one has about euthanasia. With euthanasia of course there is the element of consent, but in these cases you are really dealing with a person who is a ward of court — mentally incapacitated. How do we act? Well, we act in a negative way. Should there be complications we do not attempt any heroic measures. We see to basic needs, but avoid interventions to rescue from crises such as infections.'

The christian ethic does not hold that life should be artificially prolonged under all circumstances.[12]

(4) 'Transplants — are the donors really dead?': The whole issue of brain death was further complicated in the minds of the lay public when on Thursday evening at 8.10pm (peak viewing

time), 13 October 1980, BBC 1 devoted their Panorama programme to the subject: 'Transplants — are the donors really dead?' Six million viewers watched with astonishment and concern the case-histories of four American patients supposedly diagnosed as 'brain dead', who in fact had suffered from a reversible alteration of brain function from which they recovered to live normal lives again. Much public concern was expressed, for this was a direct challenge to the British concept of brain death. (I happened to be visiting one of the hospital wards the following morning and discussed the programme with some of our senior nursing staff. One staff nurse informed me that her brother had ripped up his kidney donor card immediately after watching the programme!) Much attention was given to the case histories; a man who had been unconscious after cardiac arrest; a woman with a drug overdose, and a man with severe accidental injuries; in all of whom brain death was reported to have been diagnosed, yet the patient recovered.

The important fact to note is that not one of these patients would have been diagnosed as 'brain dead' according to our UK criteria. Professor Bryan Jennett and Dr Christopher Pallis *et al.* clearly demonstrated in the correspondence columns of the leading medical journals and *The Times*, how extremely unfortunate it was that the BBC programme failed to make clear to the viewers that a very strict code of practice had several years previously been set up by the Royal Colleges in the UK in order to prevent any possibility of an erroneous diagnosis of brain death. Professor Jennett's maxim is extremely reassuring: 'When in doubt there is no doubt: one should not diagnose death.'[13] If the UK criteria are strictly applied the system is foolproof.

Before we go on to consider some of the salient points of the UK criteria it might be helpful to describe as simply as possible the structure of the brain and its various components emphasizing the part played by the brain stem.

The Brain And Its Structure

The brain has several levels of activity. There is the cerebrum, with its outer shell called the cortex which is the highest level of activity relating to thinking, experiences and consciousness. For this reason it is often referred to as the 'higher brain'.

There are subcortical levels of activity relating to reflex auto-
nomic and emotional responses. There are the cerebellum and
the brain stem, comprising the mid-brain, the pons and the
medulla oblongata. The brain stem is often referred to as the
'inner brain' for it controls spontaneous vegetative functions
such as swallowing, yawning and sleep-wake cycles. The pontine levels of activity modulate posture and respiration. In the
medulla area exist the vital centres of respiration, circulation
and cardiac action.

When the respiratory centre of the brain is destroyed respiration ceases and this deprives the heart of its much needed
oxygen, which in turn causes it to stop functioning. When
respiration and heart beat ceases the person is dead. However,
as we have already seen, the respirator and life support systems have changed this traditional and straightforward picture. Sophisticated technology which can now be used to
support or supplant certain vital functions have thus created
new problems in diagnosing death.

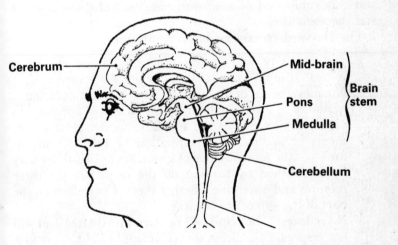

It is imperative that the diagnosis of death be incontroverti-
ble. It must be confirmed that respiration is solely an artefact
of mechanical intervention, and that nothing is done during
testing which might impede or hinder the recovery of a patient
who might be found to have partial or reversible brain
functioning. When kidney transplantation came into vogue in

the 1960s, and heart transplantation in the late 1960s, it became even more important for physicians and all concerned with the care of the patient to be able to diagnose and confirm when the brain of a mechanically supported patient had irretrievably ceased functioning. Medical concern over such vital matters led to the setting out of various guidelines which might reliably confirm permanent loss of brain function and so establish brain death. It is to these that we now turn.

Published Criteria

The best safeguard against any suspicion of error is a set of well written clear guidelines. There are at present over thirty different world-wide criteria for the diagnosis of brain death, but they differ little in their essentials.

The first official working guidelines came in *A Report of the Ad Hoc Committee of the Harvard Medical School to examine the definition of brain-death* (1968), which advocated the adoption of 'irreversible coma as a new definition of death'. The Committee was chaired by Henry Beecher, Professor of Anaesthetics, and was comprised of neurosurgeons, neurologists, lawyers and theologians.

The Harvard criteria for brain death were:

1. Unreceptivity and unresponsitivity: 'Even the most intense stimuli evoke no vocal or other response . . .'.

2. No movements or breathing: 'Observation covering a period of at least one hour by physicians is adequate to satisfy the criteria of the spontaneous muscular movements or spontaneous respiration or response to stimuli . . . the total absence of spontaneous breathing may be established by turning off the respirator for three minutes and observing whether there is any effort on the part of the subject to breathe.'

3. No reflexes: 'The pupil will be fixed and dilated and will not respond to a direct source of bright light . . . ocular movement and blinking are absent . . . there is no evidence of postural activity . . . swallowing, yawning, vocalizing are in abeyance . . .'.

4. Flat electro-encephalogram: 'Of great confirmatory value is the flat or isoelectric electro-encephalogram.'

All the above tests were to be repeated after at least 24 hours and should show no change.

Two important clarifications need to be made when referring to the original Harvard criteria:- (a) The term 'irreversible coma' led to some confusion as later it was used to describe the 'vegetative state' (see p.87). The distinction is made clear by Dr William Sweet (1978) in an editorial comment: 'It is essential that a clear distinction be made between death of the brain and a prolonged or irreversible state of coma but with some evidence of brain-related bodily function. Not only are the two terms not synonymous, but they describe two different states that do not overlap. Once a person is dead, he is no longer in coma. . . . Indeed, it is clear that the brain does not die all at once, and the "coma" sense of brain death could mean rather only the necrosis of some parts of the brain (such as the cortex). By "brain death", in the sense of "real death" we mean "total brain death", or the death of the entire brain.' Later on he makes an important observation, ' . . .It is clear that a person is not dead *unless* his brain is dead. The time-honoured criteria of stoppage of the heartbeat and circulation are indicative of death only when they persist long enough for the brain to die'.[14]

(b) Later in 1969 Henry Beecher stated that his Committee was 'unanimous in its belief that an encephalogram was not essential to a diagnosis of irreversible coma', although it could provide 'valuable supportive data'.[15]

In 1971 two neurosurgeons, A. Mohandas and Shelley N. Chou of the University of Minnesota Health Sciences Center, Minneapolis, Minnesota, USA, issued what became known as the Minnesota Criteria.[16] Briefly they can be summarized as follows.

1. No spontaneous movement.
2. No spontaneous respiration when tested for a period of 4 minutes at a time.
3. Absence of brain stem reflexes.
4. A status in which all of the findings above remain unchanged for at least 12 hours.
5. Brain death can be pronounced only if the pathological processes for states 1 to 4 above are deemed irreparable with presently available means.

It was thought an EEG was mandatory.

These two criteria much influenced thinking and practice in the UK. In 1976 came criteria proposed by the Conference of the Medical Royal Colleges and Faculties of the United Kingdom.[17] The original working party comprised doctors, nurses, and members of the legal profession; views of the main religious bodies and of health councils were also sought. Summarized they are as follows.

A. Conditions under which the diagnosis of brain death should be considered:

   1. The patient is deeply comatose.

     (a) There should be no suspicion that this state is due to depressant drugs.

     (b) Primary hypothermia as a cause of coma should have been excluded.

     (c) Metabolic and endocrine disturbances that can be responsible for or can contribute to coma should have been excluded.

   2. The patient is being maintained on a ventilator because spontaneous respiration had previously become inadequate or had ceased altogether.

     (a) Relaxant and other drugs should have been excluded as a cause of respiratory failure.

   3. There should be no doubt that the patient's condition is due to irreversible structural brain damage. The diagnosis of a disorder that can lead to brain death should have been fully established.

B. Diagnostic tests for confirmation of brain death:

   All brain stem reflexes are absent.

   1. The pupils are fixed in diameter and do not respond to sharp changes in the intensity of incident light.

   2. There is no corneal reflex.

   3. The vestibulo-ocular reflexes are absent.

   4. No motor responses within the cranial-nerve distribution can be elicited by adequate stimulation of a somatic area.

   5. There is no gag reflex or reflex response to bronchial stimulation by a suction catheter passed through the trachea.

   6. No respiratory movements occur when the patient is

disconnected from the mechanical ventilator for long enough to ensure that the arterial carbon dioxide tension rises above the threshold for stimulation of respiration.

C. Other considerations:
   1. Repetition of testing. . . . The interval between tests depends upon the progress of the patient and might be as long as 24 hours.
   2. Integrity of spinal reflexes.
   3. Confirmatory investigations. It is now widely accepted that electro-encephalography is not necessary for the diagnosis of brain death.
   4. Body temperature . . . It is recommended that it should be not less than 35°c before the diagnostic tests are carried out.
   5. Specialist opinion and the status of the doctors concerned. Only when the primary diagnosis is in doubt is it necessary to consult with a neurologist or neurosurgeon.

The decision to withdraw artificial support should be made after all the criteria above have been fulfilled and can be made by any of the following combination of doctors:
   (a) A consultant who is in charge of the case and one other doctor.
   (b) In the absence of a consultant his deputy, who should have been registered for five years or more, and who should have had adequate experience in the care of such cases and one other doctor.

In its preamble the statement affirms that 'it has been the concern of the medical profession to establish diagnostic criteria of such rigour that on their fulfilment the mechanical ventilator can be switched off, in the secure knowledge that there is no possible chance of recovery. There has been much philosophical argument about the diagnosis of death, which has throughout history been accepted as having occurred when the vital functions of respiration and circulation have ceased. With the technical ability to maintain these functions artificially, however, the dilemma of when to switch off the ventilator has been the subject of much public interest. It is agreed that permanent functional death of the brain stem constitutes brain death and that once this has occurred further artificial support is fruitless and should be withdrawn. It is good medical practice to recognize when brain death has occurred and to act accordingly, sparing relatives from the further emotional trauma of sterile hope.'

The Conference of Medical Royal Colleges and their Faculties in the UK prepared an addendum in 1979 entitled *Diagnosis of Death*, supplementing the earlier 1976 Report which made no reference to organ transplantation.[18] It examines whether death itself should be presumed to occur when brain death takes place. It states, *inter alia*, that:

2. Exceptionally, as a result of massive trauma, death occurs instantaneously or near instantaneously. Far more commonly, death is not an event, it is a process, the various organs and systems supporting the continuation of life failing and eventually ceasing altogether to function, successively and at different times.

3. . . . Since the moment that the heartbeat ceases is usually detectable with simplicity . . . it has for many centuries been accepted as the moment of death itself, without any serious attempt being made to assess the validity of this assumption. . . .

4. It is now universally accepted, by the lay public as well as by the medical profession, that it is not possible to equate death itself with cessation of the heartbeat. . . .

7. Whatever the mode of its production, brain death represents the stage at which a patient becomes truly dead, because by then all functions of the brain have permanently and irreversibly ceased. It is not difficult or illogical in any way to equate this with the concept in many religions of the departure of the spirit from the body. . . .

9. It is the conclusion of the Conference that the identification of brain death means that the patient is dead, whether or not the function of some organs, such as a heartbeat, is still maintained by artificial means.

Are these 1976 and 1979 Royal Colleges' criteria satisfactory?, I asked a number of doctors. The majority view was that they are stringent. Mr Peter Wilson asserted that

> 'they have not been challenged by a single authenticated instance of failure.'

Dr Victor Parsons thought that the criteria are getting better known and are working very well. He considered them to be

> 'absolutely, totally watertight. There may be one or two borderline cases but they are very, very few. With the practice of medicine as it is at the moment the criteria are as satisfactory as one can get.'

Professor Sir Gordon Robson considered the 1976 and 1979 Royal Colleges criteria to be most satisfactory:

> 'The criteria are based on a wide knowledge of all possibilities and they are extremely precisely worded. Since they cover everything, in some cases they could be judged as being over elaborate in the light of the clinical circumstances of individual cases. Nevertheless, they provide the highest degree of safety for every patient.'

Although these codes and guidelines have no legal sanction they have been widely accepted and may be assumed to be the official standard for the determination of brain-stem death in the United Kingdom. It will have been seen that these British criteria rely upon clinical examination only and do not use either electro-encephalography or arteriography. The use of electro-encephalography is not considered necessary for the diagnosis of brain death, for it does not help and may even confuse. For example, it may show no function in the brain in patients with recoverable brain disorders (in particular, overdose of drugs), and it may show continuing electrical activity in some patients with irreversible damage to the brain.

In his centre at Swansea, Peter Wilson informed me that it was their policy to

> 'have (preferably repeated) EEG recordings in patients with clinical brain death. This is not, however, orthodox or widespread in UK neurosurgical centres. There are

perfectly valid technical and pragmatic reasons for this. We have seen no clinically brain-dead patient whose EEG was not iso-electric.

We foresee that future technological refinements will enable other reliable non-evasive bedside tests to be done to corroborate the clinical diagnosis, e.g. tests of cerebral circulation; gross cerebral metabolic dissolution.'

Professor J.K. Mason very much doubted whether an electro-encephalogram would add any further support to the criteria, but thought that

'relatives should have a right to ask for it if it will set their minds at rest.'

A similar opinion was expressed by Professor Peter Morris:

'I do not feel that the EEG does add anything to the British criteria of brain death. However, it may provide emotional support on occasion.'

It is not very sensible to *insist* on it, Professor Sir Gordon Robson explained,

'because although an electro-encephalogram has some diagnostic uses I would hate to be diagnosed as "brain dead" on the basis of having a flat tracing. A "flat" tracing does not mean brain death and it cannot of itself be regarded as being confirmatory of the diagnosis established by the recommended tests. It is therefore not part of the criteria of diagnosis.'

The Royal Colleges state that testing the function of the whole brain is as irrelevant as testing the function of the liver; the clinical question is whether the patient has any chance of recovery.[19] The criteria try to avoid the problem of intoxication as a potential cause of brain death by the exclusion of cases in which the diagnosis of a destructive brain lesion is in doubt. Again the criteria allow for as short a period as seems reasonable for the diagnosis instead of specifying a time period. It is clear that they are designed to make the likelihood of erroneous diagnosis as close to impossible as human fallibility allows.

All these UK criteria are reproduced in the *Code of Practice*

for the Transplantation of Cadaveric Organs. The code was orig-
inally published in 1979 by the Health Departments.[20] The
later revised version (1983) contains no significant changes,
but some sections have been clarified. Mr Kenneth Clark,
Minister of Health, in a written Commons reply after the
Government had issued the revised code of practice, gave the
assurance that 'there is not the slightest chance, when the
code is followed, that organs will be removed for transplantation from someone who is not dead in every sensible meaning of the term. It is a tragedy that fears of that kind have cost
hundreds of operations that might have returned patients to
happy and full lives'. In this second edition of the Code of
Practice a revised checklist has been agreed which itemizes
the reconditions and tests, each one to be checked by each
doctor on two occasions. As Professor Bryan Jennett con-
fidently asserted:

> 'There is no other procedure in medicine that has such
> stringent safeguards as these and there should be no
> question of clinical error'.

It is made plain that the criteria give recommended guidelines
rather than rigid rules, and that it is for the doctors at the
bedside to decide when the patient is dead.

From Brain Death to Brain-Stem Death

It will be seen that all the criteria for brain death assume that
death of the *brain stem* is equivalent to the death of the person.
The brain often dies in a gradual and progressive way; usually
the cortex dies first, then the mid-brain and then finally the
brain-stem. As the brain stem maintains all vital functions,
being responsible for breathing, heart-beat and consciousness,
once it is destroyed all our functions cease. However, this
transition from a cardiac-based death to a cerebral-orientated
death has led to a failure among some physicians to agree
upon the criteria that are necessary to establish the death of
the brain.[21]

This next step forward, of death of the brain-stem being
seen as the necessary and sufficient component of whole brain
death, created one of the main areas of confusion in the whole
discussion on the subject of brain death. There are some who
consider death as 'dissolution of the whole organism'; in other

words where death is seen as 'total body death'. Others require the destruction of the higher brain and the brain-stem. There is a reluctance on the part of such physicians to take the step from brain-stem death to total brain death. Dr Christopher Pallis (1983) summarizes the argument thus:[22] 'The irreversible cessation of heartbeat and respiration imply death *of the patient as a whole*. They do not necessarily imply the immediate death of *every cell in the body*. The irreversible cessation of brain-stem function implies death *of the brain as a whole*. It does not necessarily imply the immediate death of *every cell in the brain*.' He concludes by stating that 'if we accept the concept of brain-stem death it might be wise to change the words we use and no longer speak of "brain death" when we mean "brain stem death"'.

The brain-stem is, as it were, the 'Clapham Junction' through which all 'trains' travel, and it maintains all the relevant 'signals'. Once it is destroyed no 'trains' (vital functions) can operate. Those who support the 'total brain death' concept are not prepared to diagnose death until the upper brain as well as the brain-stem have lost all their activity and function. Proponents of this viewpoint wish to confirm the cessation of function in each and every one of the brain cells so that no electrical activity is evident before certifying brain death. But as cells with low oxygen requirements (in skin and the matrix of bone) may remain alive for variable periods after the heart has permanently ceased to beat, 'putrefaction would be the only criterion relevant to such a concept of biological death'.

Professor Jennett explained it further:

> 'I think one has to try to put across that death is a process; that it doesn't overcome the entire body simultaneously. Indeed, lay observation teaches this — you can take skin grafts, you can take bones out and put them in the bank, you can take kidneys out. There are different periods of survival for different organs and tissues. Now the brain is the most delicate of organs. It would only last a few minutes like that, but the skin would last, I'm not sure how long. One has to get away from the notion of death as something which happens in an instant, which, of course, it very seldom may do. Normally death is a

process and this is what the slogan means about "the organism as a whole".'

Discontinuing The Ventilator

When a patient is considered to be brain dead the Conference of Medical Royal Colleges and their faculties in the UK recommend, as we have already noted, that the diagnosis should be made by two medical practitioners who have expertise in this field (one consultant and the other a consultant or senior registrar; they will usually be neurosurgeons, neurologists, intensive care physicians, or anaesthetists). After various clinical tests have been carried out and a declaration of brain-stem death has been confirmed (in writing and signed) the patient is declared dead and the family and relatives informed. The patient may then be disconnected from the ventilator, a procedure that should be performed by a doctor and not delegated to a member of the nursing staff, however senior the nurse may be. The death certificate can be issued while the patient still has a beating heart and ventilation is being continued, when donation of organs is planned. Legally speaking the time of death is when brain death is confirmed, not at some later time when the heart stops.

'The instructions in my unit are quite clear', Professor Jennett informed me, 'that whenever possible the death certificate should be given to the relatives at this point of time.'

(The Code of Practice: *Cadaveric Organs for Transplantation*, states (p. 12) that 'the time of death should be recorded as the time when death was conclusively established, not . . . when artificial ventilation is withdrawn, or the heartbeat ceases'.)

As there is a great deal of misunderstanding and sensationalizing of this issue, for example, by the use of such expressions as 'discontinuing life support', 'pulling the plug', it needs to be emphasized that when the doctor disconnects the ventilator he is not withdrawing treatment to allow the patient to die; he is ceasing to keep ventilating a body already dead. As Professor Bryan Jennett aptly put it:

'The doctor is not withdrawing treatment and allowing

someone to die, but ceasing to do something useless to someone who is already dead.'

A diagnosis of brain death should never be considered as a justification for switching off the ventilator *prematurely*. In no sense are doctors 'acting as God'; they are not withholding something from someone who otherwise would die, neither are they practising euthanasia. It is because the patient has been declared dead, and for *no other reason*, that the ventilator is 'switched off'. There can be no point in artificial prolongation of life beyond the state at which recovery, or even partial recovery, becomes impossible. No doctor has the obligation to keep a person alive at all costs.

If the ventilator is not disconnected until the heart stops spontaneously the extremities of the body may commence to decompose, and all the dignity of dying is lost and the grief of the family extended. Hopes are being raised in circumstances where there is no hope. The death of the individual should take place under the most humane conditions not only for the sake of the family but also for members of the nursing staff. Death should always be seen as a truly human act, dignified and sacred.

Conclusions

There is no formal legal definition of death in the UK and the majority of doctors agree that such legislation would not be definitive and binding. I asked whether a more specific and objectively stated definition of death was necessary for moral and legal purposes, and, was there a case for a statute concerning the occurrence of death which might possibly remove all doubts in the minds of both doctors and public? Mr Peter Wilson gave an emphatic

> 'No! An overly-rigid legalistic definition of death will do nothing to strengthen existing criteria. There is only one criterion of death that would satisfy *every* doubter, and that is *decomposition*. I am told that a few consultants *have* actually waited for this to occur before switching off a ventilator! Incredible! Inhuman?'

A similar opinion was expressed by Professor J. K. Mason:

> 'No. Not so long as you use the term brain-stem death,

because then all is defined. The trouble with a statute is that it can never be all embracing and the law will almost certainly lag behind medical technology. A statute might, therefore, be counter-productive; at worst, it could be the basis for unjustifiable litigation. It is important to realize that judicial approval has already been given to the concepts of brain-stem death (HMAdv v. Finlayson: R v. Malcherek), but the judges were anxious not, themselves, to attempt a definition of death. Rather, they determined that removal from a ventilator could be good medical practice, thereby leaving the doctor unconstrained in coming to a clinical decision.'

If there was to be legislation, what form did Professor Mason think it should take?

'The essential thing is that a statute, which I believe is unnecessary, should be no more than an enabling act. That is, it should "enable doctors to certify death in accordance with accepted medical practice at the time, irrespective of the fact that the heart and lungs are functioning by virtue of extracorporeal support." What it must *not* do is to attempt to lay down diagnostic criteria.'

Professor Peter Morris considered that the definition of death is best left where it is now; namely the patient is dead when the doctor says the patient is dead. He maintained that

'to provide a statue concerning a legal definition of death would provide enormous problems both for the lawyer as well as the doctor, and would shift responsibility for defining death from doctors to lawyers, which would be unsatisfactory.'

We are not, of course, as litigious or legalistic a society as America, explained Professor Jennett.

'In America there has been a lot of pressure for brain death statute. The present situation is that about twenty-six of the States there do have such a brain death law; the first being in 1970 in Kansas. I don't sense there is any pressure here in this country — we don't have the appetite for the law here that America has.'

It was the opinion of Mr Michael Bewick that

> 'if you make it legal or put it down in the statutes, then
> you have got to make some provision for continual
> changes in scientific method and continual advances in
> scientific studies.'

Each case is considered individually, and to formulate
inflexible rules would be alien to the practice of medicine.
There must be an element of judgement and rarely is one rule
applicable in every circumstance. The task of determining the
exact time of death lies in the province of the physician rather
than in the hands of the law.[23]

The concept of brain-stem death as a determining factor in
the death of a patient seems to be acceptable to most religious
traditions. The Orthodox Jewish response to death being
pronounced on brain-related criteria is based on biblical and
talmudic doctrines. In the rabbinical literature it is the ability
to breathe independently which is the 'esse' of life, and
considered of more importance than the beating of the heart.
'And the Lord God formed man of the dust of the ground, and
breathed into his nostrils the breath of life; and man became a
living soul' (Genesis 2.7). The Code of Laws was well aware
that the state resembling cerebral death for beheading was a
commonplace occurrence of the time; the agonizing cries of 'a
decapitated man were looked upon as the aftermath of death,
and not as evidence of life. Thus, cerebral death is readily
understood as a physiological state analogous to decapitation;
respiration, a critical criterion of life, is lost as well as the
higher integrative functions, so the pronunciation of death
may be made on biblical standards. The fact that heart action
persists is not consequential since its cessation is considered a
cause, not evidence, of death.'[24]

In the Anglican and Roman Catholic Churches there is no
official authoritative pronouncement, but some of their leading moral theologians have generally accepted a concept of
death based on brain function. The traditional teaching of the
Roman Catholic Church is that the moment of real death is
based upon the time of departure of the soul from the body.
But as this cannot possibly be an objective phenomenon it
must be related to physically measurable signs defining

apparent death. Pope Pius XII, making reference to patients who are terminally unconscious, stated that 'we can refer to the usual concept of separation . . . of the soul from the body; but on the practical level, one needs to be mindful of the connotation of the terms "body" and "separation". . . . As to the pronouncement of death in certain particular cases, the answer cannot be inferred from religious and moral principles, and consequently, it is an aspect lying outside the competence of the Church.'[25] Modern Roman Catholic theologians seem to confirm that the arguments for the equation of the total death of the person with brain death are perfectly valid, and that once the fact of brain death has been established, the person is dead.[26]

One of the main religious concerns is that patients who are victims of brain-stem death, together with their families and relatives, be treated with the utmost dignity and respect, competence and compassion. There should be the firm assurance in the minds of the lay public that the best possible standard of technical and professional practice be observed, and that no *premature* termination of possible therapy be carried out under the guise of declaring brain-stem death.

The author wishes to acknowledge his gratitude to Bryan Jennett, Professor of Neurosurgery, Institute of Neurological Sciences, University of Glasgow, for commenting upon and reading through the original draft of this chapter for medical accuracy.

4

Handicapped Infants: To Live or Let Die?

The technological scope of neonatal medicine over the past decades with its advances in intensive care, drug therapy, anaesthesia, surgery, and transfusion techniques, has enabled paediatricians to save the lives of very low birth weight newborn babies. Some of these have congenital defects and the majority of them would have died a generation ago. Much has been done to alleviate and improve the quality of life of severely handicapped infants, enabling them to become fully integrated members of the community. The main work has been with very low birth weight babies who have no congenital defect but all of whose systems are immature, especially the lungs and liver. Yesterday's heroic efforts have become today's routine procedures. This newly found capability to save young lives, in which paediatricians, obstetricians and others take justifiable pride, has brought with it a trail of complex ethical questions and problems which at present are the concern not only of the lay public but also the medical world at large.

In the past when paediatricians were faced with newborn infants suffering from severe congenital defects they did their best to deal with the handicaps with the treatments available. There seemed an unwritten code between doctors and midwives not to hurry a badly deformed or severely handicapped infant into life. At a time when shunts and other surgical methods of treatment were unknown, the majority of the neonates died and there was no ethical dilemma, for no choice had to be made. Before the development of treatment for spina bifida was introduced forty per cent of infants born with meningomyelocele in London were born dead.[1]

Such concern centres around the 'sanctity of life' and 'quality of life' ethic. What quality of life are we saving? Should the life of every newborn infant be saved no matter how severe the handicap or defect may be? To what extent, if any, should the assessments of the potential quality of life influence decisions to treat or not to treat? If such decisions are to be made, who is to be responsible for making them? If certain handicapped infants are to be allowed to die, where is the line to be drawn? Such decisions to withhold or withdraw treatment are both intricate and complex. What such agonizing moral, ethical, and legal decisions mean to those who are actively engaged in this field of medicine is highlighted for us in the words of one such surgeon: 'Life is the most precious thing in the world. Is it so to the individual born without a brain capable of comprehending existence? Is life worthwhile when burdened with deformities that make social seclusion necessary. . . . Maybe it is. . . . Our duty as doctors is crystal clear — to preserve life. And yet when looking at a hopeless little mass of deformed humanity, compassion wrestles with duty.'[2]

We can the more readily place these ethical issues into perspective if we understand some of the more common major handicaps with which the majority of paediatricians and obstetricians have to deal.

Spina Bifida

Out of some 110,000 live births there are approximately 2,000 babies born each year with spina bifida, Down's syndrome, anencephaly and other deformities. Spina bifida literally means 'split spine', and it is the commonest major disabling abnormality apparent at birth. It is a defect in the spinal column in which one or more of the bones which form the backbone fail to form properly and so leave a gap or split. The cause is at present unknown and as yet there is no cure although much valuable research is being done. The condition arises in the very early stages of development probably before the mother realizes she is pregnant. The overall incidence of spina bifida in the UK is in the region of 2.5 per 1,000 live births, with a higher incidence in S. W. Scotland, South Wales (five per 1,000) and Ireland (eight per 1,000). Its most common form and also its most serious is myelomeningocele (also called meningomyelocele). Part of the spinal cord itself may be damaged or not properly formed, and as a result there is always some degree of paralysis and frequently there is incontinence. Eighty per cent of babies with spina bifida also have hydrocephalus (commonly known as 'water on the brain'). The main physical symptom is a large head which if not treated will get larger due to the build-up of fluid. Brain damage occurs as a result of the pressure caused by the excess fluid. Formerly the majority of babies born with this defect died in the first weeks of birth from meningitis, infections and hydrocephalus. In 1958 it became possible by introducing a shunt to drain the excess fluid into the blood on the peritoneal cavity of the abdomen, and so control the hydrocephalus. Because of improved methods of surgical treatment to close the lesion, deal with incontinence and correct orthopaedic problems, many more children have survived. New antibiotics have also been developed to combat infection.

Down's Syndrome

This is the commonest form of mental handicap and is sometimes called 'mongolism'. It is a condition which affects one in every 600 babies. Its cause remains unknown and there is no cure. Down's syndrome (so called for it was first described by Dr John Langdon Down in 1866) arises from a chance abnormality in the chromosomes, which are minute particles in the nuclei of cells that constitute the body. Half of a person's forty-six chromosomes per cell are inherited from mother, and half from father. A baby with this syndrome acquires an extra chromosome at conception. There are certain physical characteristics and it is often possible to recognize the condition in the first few weeks of life or even at birth. The baby is short in stature, with the skull round and flat at the rear. Hands and feet are thick and square; fingers and toes short and stubby. The eyes have an upward and outward slant (hence the term 'mongolism'). There may be abnormalities in the heart and circulation, and the brain and nervous system are poorly developed. Prior to World War Two many Down's children lived in institutions, but, with the development of family caring and antibiotics, life expectancy has improved and the majority now survive into adult life. Nevertheless, rather more than a third die during the first five years of life. The question 'to live or let die' should not relate to any Down's syndrome baby.

Although the above seem to be the main examples of increasing numbers of infant abnormalities, there are of course others which although less common are nevertheless by no means less tragic (cerebral agenesis and anencephaly etc). These present similar moral, ethical as well as medical problems.

To Live or Let Die?

The whole subject of the care of handicapped infants came to the forefront as a result of two recent incidences, both of which concerned babies born with Down's syndrome.

1. On 25 June 1980, John Pearson was born in Derby City Hospital, and was found at birth to be suffering from Down's syndrome. He was rejected by his parents. Dr Leonard Arthur, a consultant paediatrician, prescribed 'nursing care' only for baby John. Regular doses of the drug DF118 were also prescribed. On 1 July 1980, John died. On 5 February 1981 Dr Arthur was charged with the murder of baby Pearson. He stood for trial before Mr Justice Farquharson at Leicester Crown Court on 13 October 1981. The charge of murder was reduced to attempted murder, and Dr Arthur was eventually acquitted at the end of the trial on 5 November 1981.

It is important to record that infant John was a Down's syndrome baby *without* any complications. At the post-mortem examination there was evidence of some damage to the heart, lungs and brain, but apparently this was not known to Dr Arthur when his original decision was taken.

2. A small infant, named Alexandra, was born in July 1981 at Queen Charlotte's Hospital, London, with Down's syndrome. Shortly after her birth an operation was needed to remove an intestinal obstruction. Without the operation life expectancy was approximately one week. Because of the physical handicap and all that it might involve, her parents refused to give permission for the operation to be performed. They believed, it was stated in the national press, that 'God or nature had given the child a way out'. Medical opinion expressed firmly that the operation should be performed, and the local Hammersmith and Fulham Council was informed to this effect and Alexandra was made a ward of court on 31 July when she was

three days old. The judge, after hearings held in the Appeal Court, ordered the surgeons to proceed with the operation, and the following day, 6 August, this was successfully carried out at Hammersmith Hospital.

Very naturally press, television and radio covered the story with typical thoroughness, and on the whole the general reaction supported the decision of the Court, which was seen to have the best interests of the child at heart. Yet much of the medical world was divided. Many resented the court's interference in what they considered to be solely a parental and medical decision.

These two cases illustrate both ethical and legal implications, and they bring the whole process of decision-making as well as society's attitude towards the physically and/or mentally handicapped into question. Should the life of a child depend upon whether the parents want it or not? Are doctors to be the sole arbiters of such agonizing life-death decisions? Should the law be involved at all?

Screening Procedures

One approach to the problem is so-called 'prevention'. Prenatal screening is now available and consists of various tests which are likely to detect malformation, mainly a neural tube defect (NTD) such as spina bifida and Down's syndrome, in an expected baby. In tests for neural tube defects a sample of the mother's blood is checked for alpha-feto-protein (AFP), which is a protein which passes into the amniotic fluid and into the mother's blood from the baby. It comes from the exposed choroid plexus in the brain and spinal cord of the baby, and its function is to form brain fluid. This test is offered at 16–19 weeks, in which 16 weeks is considered the optimum time. Simultaneously an ultra-sound scan should be carried out. If the results of these tests appear to be unfavourable an amniocentesis is performed. In this screening procedure a needle is inserted through the wall of the mother's abdomen, through the muscle of the uterus, and then into the amniotic sac. A sample of the amniotic fluid is drawn off and checked for AFP. The test for Down's syndrome always requires an amniocentesis, when a clear sample of the amniotic fluid is required to ensure the fetal cells can be cultured.

It is claimed that after the sixteenth to seventeenth week of pregnancy all cases of anencephaly and nine out of ten cases of severe neural-tube malformation compatible with life can be detected early enough for termination of pregnancy to be carried out. Professor Stuart Campbell, King's College Hospital, London, who runs one of the most sophisticated screening programmes for pregnant women, has stated that he has had only five mothers out of three hundred who have decided to keep their baby when they discovered it was seriously handicapped.

Is abortion justified when a fetus is diagnosed as abnormal? For a number of people under no circumstances is abortion acceptable; to them the sanctity of life is of paramount importance. There are others who would concede that a justified exception may be made when the fetus is threatening the life of the mother. Some would argue that selective abortion is merely expediting mother nature, for a large number of pregnancies abort spontaneously (some authorities place this as high as seventy-eight per cent), and a high proportion of these aborted fetuses are abnormal. They argue that as nature obviously intends to eliminate the seriously abnormal why should not man be deemed justified in assisting her.[3] Section 4 of the Abortion Act (1967) states that an abortion may be legally carried out where 'there is substantial risk that if the child were born it would suffer from such physical or mental abnormalities as to be seriously handicapped'.

These screening tests are obviously not performed on every pregnant woman but only on those where there appears a high risk of a handicapped child being born to them. Consequently they will only 'prevent' the birth of some five per cent of all spina bifida babies. Results can be made available within a few days of the test being performed.

The BMA *Handbook of Medical Ethics* (1981) stipulates that 'in considering the financial implications, the doctor should remember that it will be some time before the cost of the screening programme is offset by the benefits accrued from earlier diagnosis of the disease'. For this reason it seems best that resources should be concentrated in a relatively small number of units throughout each area. The Handbook also refers to some of the ethical dilemmas of presymptomatic screening in general, due to the fact that 'screening could reveal many sick persons who do not at present seek medical help' (p. 31).

Used by experienced and highly skilled staff the procedure of amniocentesis is comparatively safe, but there are certain degrees of risk involved to mother and baby. The potential hazards are inducing a miscarriage, immediate injury to the baby, infection, and longer term hazards to the baby. Although there are risks they are small provided amniocentesis is done under conditions mentioned above. Fortunately most of these hazards are correctable.[4]

Recent studies have shown how help can be given to mothers at risk of having a defective baby by prescribing vitamins and nutrient supplements before and during the first weeks of pregnancy.[5] Further technological advances will probably enable obstetricians to diagnose and prevent more fetal abnormalities.

Genetic Counselling

Another important feature of preventive procedures is that of genetic counselling. Professor Peter Harper (1981) defines its principles as 'the process by which patients or relatives at risk of a disorder that may be hereditary are advised of the consequences of the disorder, the probability of developing and transmitting it and of the ways in which this may be prevented or ameliorated'.[6] Such a definition synthesizes three basic factors: the diagnostic which enables sound advice to be proferred, the estimation of the risks in given situations, and a supportive role giving to those counselled an accurate knowledge of the various supportive measures available. Genetic counselling is non-directive with an emphasis on informing clients and not making decisions for them.

The counsellor will ensure that individuals have the facts to enable them to reach their own decisions. About fifty per cent of those who seek counselling help are parents of handicapped infants or of children who have other damage of unknown origin in which genes may or may not have played a part. They will obviously seek advice as to whether subsequent children might be affected, and also be desirous to know what resources are available to help them care for their existing child. Others who are prospective parents and aware of relatives affected with an inherited disorder may wish for more information relating to the disease, and the likelihood of its occurrence both in themselves and their children. Parents are enabled to plan for the future care of a handicapped offspring and also helped in the acceptance of the child into their own personal lives, their families and the community at large. All such counselling interviews are naturally kept within the strictest confidence and the personal beliefs, attitudes and values of the client respected.

Decision-making in many instances is by no means an easy or straightforward matter, and must ultimately be made by the respective individuals guided by their understanding of the facts and by their conscience.

Some helpful criteria have been outlined in the WCC (World Council of Churches) Study Encounter (1974):

(a) The severity of the genetic disorder and its effect on the possibility of a meaningful life, or the probability of death: i.e. if death in infancy is certain, some parents will prefer that to abortion.

(b) The physical, emotional and economic impact on family (parents and other children) and society.

(c) The availability of adequate medical management and of special educational and other facilities.

(d) The reliability of diagnosis and the predictability of the expression of the genetic disorder involved, both in degree and variability in manifestation of symptoms.

(e) The recognition that an individual genetically defective in one respect may be superior in others, and in fact may compensate (or even overcompensate) for his defect by development of other abilities or talents.[7] Genetic counselling helps them to understand the choices open to them and provides them with a context into which to fit the dictates of their own conscience. It is also helpful for parents and prospective parents to receive psychological and spiritual support as required.

Such counselling should take place before conception and continue during the prenatal period. At present the majority of those who seek help already have one defective infant. High-risk relatives pose a problem, for it may be clear from the family history that there are other persons within the family circle who are of high-risk category. Should they be told? Would such telling be an invasion of privacy? These are complex situations and the course of action depends much upon circumstances. One of the main standards of genetic counselling is simplicity, and principles should be emphasized rather than mathematical statistics or percentages proferred.

Guidelines

Some helpful guideline procedures for decision-making with infants born with meningomyelocele have been drawn up by Professor John Lorber (1975) of Sheffield.[8] Prior to the 1960s it was rare for infants suffering from myelomeningocele to undergo surgery. The survival rate was estimated to be five to ten per cent, and those who did survive were severely handicapped, not only physically but also intellectually. By the 1960s, Lorber states that it was difficult for any doctor not to refer babies for surgery, and for a surgeon not to operate for fear of adverse criticism.

A combined team of paediatric and orthopaedic surgeons, paediatricians and supporting services, was set up at Sheffield in 1959 but the results of such aggressive surgical policy, when, between 1959 and 1968, 848 infants were treated from the first day of life, were later seen to be far from beneficial. Only fifty per cent of the babies survived in spite of all the care, innumerable operations and medical treatment. The most frequent causes of later deaths were shunt complications and progressive renal disease. Only six survivors (1.4 per cent) had no handicaps; a further seventy-three (17.2 per cent) had what might be termed 'moderate handicap in a spina bifida context'. Of those who survived, 345 (or over eighty per cent) had severe multi-system physical defects.

The effect on families was devastating at the time, for it was obviously much harder for parents to lose their child after several years of devoted care and after many operations, than it would have been had they lost their child soon after birth. According to Lorber many parents aged prematurely through constant anxiety and recurrent crises. The upbringing of brothers and sisters suffered and some families broke up. Perhaps worst of all, many potentially normal lives were never started because their parents did not dare to have other children.

After the vast experience gained as a result of this non-selective approach over a period of some ten years, the Sheffield team decided in 1971 to attempt to find suitable criteria for selective treatment for handicapped infants. The social background of the infant was to be taken into account, and the main object of selection was 'not to avoid treating those who would survive with severe handicaps'. The suggested guidelines stipulate that 'it is essential once the decision not to operate has been reached, that nothing should be done which might prolong the infant's survival, but every infant should be given normal nursing care, and should be protected against suffering. They should be fed on demand. Analgesics, sedatives or anti-convulsants may be given as needed. They should be nursed in an ordinary cot with a simple dressing on the spina bifida. Tube-feeding, the administration of oxygen or resuscitation is forbidden. Infections are not treated with antibiotic drugs.'

It should be stressed that John Lorber, who informed me that his views had not changed since he first drew up the guidelines, does not see his criteria as all-embracing or as a solution to the problem. He acknowledges that 'everyone realizes that the solution offered by "selection" is not a good one. There is no "good" solution to a desperate insoluble problem, merely a "least bad solution" which is being offered.'[9]

Selective Treatment

The above criteria are now broadly adopted in the majority of the main paediatric units throughout the country. They gained the support of a working party set up by the Newcastle Regional Hospital Board (1973) chaired by the then Bishop of Durham. The Report outlines two fundamental principles about the ethical problems involved in the selective treatment of spina bifida which have opposing conclusions, namely, the estimate of the balance of suffering and happiness for those concerned, and the assertion that human life is sacred. The group put forward three important circumstances which call for the closest consideration:

(a) The *qualitative* element: what level of living will medical intervention offer to a child?

(b) The *hardship* element: what burdens will be placed on parents by the permanent care of a severely handicapped child?

(c) The *social* element: how strained are medical resources by the following of a non-selective policy?

The conclusions reached by the members of the working-party were that 'the doctor has no ethical obligation to treat cases in which the likely benefits are very dubious. Thus in the present state of medical knowledge the policy of selection for the treatment of spina bifida is in our opinion justified. We believe that the list of initial adverse criteria, set out by Lorber, provides a sufficient basis for such selection, but we recognize that these criteria change and should be subject to constant scrutiny in the light of medical advance and the conflict of ethical principles. . . . The long-term aims of medical research in this field must be to recognize the causes of these abnormalities and to remove them.'[10]

A number of physicians and surgeons are concerned about the ethical implications of the principle of selection, and in particular see the withdrawal of antibiotics as an act of negligence. Others would qualify this latter view point, for they consider that the withdrawal of antibiotics can show true care if to give them would prolong dying rather than enrich living.

There are doctors who adjudge that withholding treatment, and in some instances sedating, withholding food and only giving water, to a handicapped infant, amounts to killing the baby and as such is a criminal offence (see p.123)[11]. There is much evidence available to show that the practice of allowing 'hopeless' babies to die in this way is now widespread. Recent documentary television programmes[12] seem to bear this out, as well as an editorial in the *British Medical Journal* (1981), written by an anonymous paediatrician who reveals that in the absence of any strong parental desire to rear a severely spina bifida and hydrocephalic child, the baby is given 'careful and loving nursing, water to satisfy thirst, and increasing doses of sedation'.[13] A recent Report, *Euthanasia and Clinical Practice* (1982), also alleges that evidence is becoming increasingly available to the general public that involuntary euthanasia of certain newborn babies is a systematic rather than an occasional occurrence in certain paediatric units.[14]

Some physicians are troubled about those who are un-treated 'survivors'. Although according to Lorber ninety per cent of untreated cases are dead by their first birthday, a number live on for years and their quality of life seems worse than if they had been treated initially. Given the choice of treating or not treating, these paediatricians therefore feel obliged to give maximum treatment to all. It should be made clear that it does not necessarily follow that if surgeons oper-ate on a spina bifida child the child will live and if they do not operate he will die.

There are paediatricians who argue that in a selection policy there is always the risk of error which would, of course, endanger those infants who may live when it had been orig-inally considered they would die. In order to avoid such risks, since there can be no certainty which would die, they feel obliged to give every child optimal care.[15]

A number of doctors seem reluctant to deal with these agonizing and complex life-death issues. Yet, as an editorial in the *British Medical Journal*, 1981, makes plain: 'Problems of this kind cannot be ducked by doctors and nurses; they have to choose between treatment and non-treatment, sedation or not, and on the basis of a set of rational, consistent criteria rather than individual ad hoc judgements.'[16] Decision-making cannot be abdicated; some kind of standards have to be used in deciding whether it is advisable to continue treatment in severe cases. Some find it extremely difficult, for example, to 'give up'; an attitude which seems so contrary to the tenets of their medical training. For paediatricians who have to deal so much with the beginning of life, it must be no easy decision to accept death as an inevitable part of life. To adopt hard and fast rules — every child to be operated on, or vice versa — is a policy which is somewhat easier for some to accept, for it evades many of the ethical and moral issues about decision-making. But Duff and Campbell (1979) make the interesting point that it is the very agonizing and heart-searching involved in facing up to these problems and choices that confers the best protection on infants and their families from caprice and tyranny of sometimes cruel technology.[17] The failure to face the issues involved may well constitute an abandonment of patients in times of greatest need.

Decisions should never be arbitrarily or hastily made and it is always helpful if they can be widely shared. The more parental support the better for all the family. Professor Peter Gray emphasized the part that siblings can play in the decision-making, particularly older children:

> 'They often have a viewpoint different from the parents and see things in a better light. By being brought into the discussions they are being made co-carers of their brother or sister. They don't really regard their brother/sister as somebody with say, cerebral palsy — it's their brother or sister. Siblings can be extremely helpful in accepting a handicapped child into the family. They will bond with him or her, to use the modern term, easily, whereas the parents may be inclined to reject the child. The acceptance by the siblings will often encourage or place a moral responsibility upon the parents to do likewise.'

In the hospital it is often junior doctors and senior nurses who are in constant and intimate contact with young parents and babies, and they have to share many of the family's emotional fears and apprehensions. In the community general practitioners together with their social workers will have an understanding of the family background. Contact with the home doctor at this stage can often make a vast difference to the relationship of the family and the care of the parents and siblings later. Hospital chaplains and parish priests have much to contribute to the counselling of families when faced with such heart-rending decisions. It was encouraging to hear from Dr Hugh Jolly that

> 'obviously my chaplains are very much involved. I think it's possible to help with the dying as it is to help with the curing. I'm constantly saying that doctors have to be as highly trained in death as in life, and that the whole concept of the ongoing work after the death of whoever it might be is part of a doctor's job. He then determines whether the appropriate person for the ongoing work is the priest, the social worker, or the health visitor, or whoever. I think this wretched thing of doctors all being

trained to *cure* — this is their great problem. I'm always interested that there is only one letter different in terms of to *care*. Nurses are trained to care and we've got to train doctors to care as well. Hopefully they are improving but, by God, they've got a long way to go!'

Dr Janet Goodall also advocates:

'Parents seeking spiritual strength should be allowed opportunity to seek advice from moral or spiritual directors such as the hospital chaplain or family minister, and may clearly find inspiration from a personal trust in God. Humanly speaking, however, there is no escape from the fact that only specialist doctors have genuine understanding both of the pathology and of the practical pros and cons under discussion.'

The first and most important person to be considered in every decision making is the handicapped infant himself, and this is an aspect of the problem rightly emphasized by Ralph Evans and Janet Goodall:

'We must consider the questions — Whose suffering? What means and to which end? What kind of life? . . . It is possible to solve our own problems by perpetuating in the life of another an even greater one. While we fully support the concept of reverence for human life, we clearly distinguish between *cure* — or attempt at it — and *care* . . . Even if our heroic measures could save a life, we should first consider whether it would also take a hero to go on living it'.[18]

In those instances where the handicap is extremely severe the decision may be reached with general and ready agreement. In others the predicament is desperate and soul-searching, as Janet Goodall stated:

'To decide what is the right course for each infant, whether obviously handicapped or with a potentially handicapping condition, is what constitutes a paediatrician's dilemma. What could be done is not necessarily what should be done. Know-how must be harnessed to wisdom. We must not equate reverence for technical

competence with reverence for life itself, yet neither must
we try to deny the problem by bringing it to an abrupt
end.'

There may often be temptation to 'hold on', in the hope and
expectation that the infant will contact an infection which
may eventually bring about a merciful death. One of the
major problems is the uncertainty about prognosis, for it is
extremely difficult to assess with precision neurological potential in a handicapped child. This concern was expressed by Dr
Jack Insley:

> 'It is a worry because I don't think one can always be
> absolutely certain. One can only have a sort of feeling as
> a result of the way things are going. It is difficult to be
> always absolutely precise, and generally, of course, one
> would come down on the side of caution and not try and
> take risks.'

The problem was further elaborated by Dr Janet Goodall:

> 'Our dilemma is how (and whether) to forecast the likely
> outcome of active intervention, and then whether (and
> how) to intervene. We could simply settle for being
> skilled technicians, inflexibly insisting on intensive care
> for each child regardless of the consequences. Yet we also
> have a responsibility to look at the end from the begin-
> ning — to use our skills with judgement. Perhaps the
> greatest dilemma of all is whether the new technology
> has outmoded the old ethical standards and if so, what to
> put in their place.'

There are many 'grey areas' in which the physician and
others concerned have to draw on their own resources of
sensitivity, love and concern, rather than on any rigid scientific
standards, or firm social and ethical guidelines. The division
between what is technically possible and what is humanely
desirable has to be defined as clearly as possible in the given
circumstances. There can be few spheres of research and
development in which there are wider differences of opinion
on how far what is possible can be equated with what is
worthwhile. As one doctor put it:

'Almost always we are dealing with shades of grey rather than black or white. I talk with the family and listen to what they are saying between the lines as well as what they are saying overtly. Sometimes one hears some little remark which indicates that they are against heroic measures. At other times one hears pleading, "Isn't there *anything* more you can do?", encouragement to take the more drastic course. At any rate, I take into account the family's circumstances and their wishes, but then I make the recommendation.'

Both treatment and non-treatment procedures can constitute unsatisfactory and tormenting dilemmas for everyone concerned, especially for the handicapped infant and family. One can only sympathize and express concern and understanding for those upon whom such soul-searching decisions rest. It is only those personally involved who are able fully to appreciate the mental, emotional, and often spiritual agony suffered. In this respect an extremely important point was made by Dr Jolly:

'One's got to be very clear that as well as the enormous distress of the parents there is the enormous distress of the professionals. I don't think enough has been written or said about this. We've got to be looking at their needs as well.'

Omission — Commission

Is withholding treatment ethically different from terminating life? Is there a moral difference between 'killing' and 'letting die'; between 'acts' and 'omissions'? There is considerable debate among philosophers over these questions. The distinction between 'act' and 'omission' has been defined as follows: 'To act is intentionally ("at will") to *bring about* or *prevent* a *change* in the world (in nature). By this definition, to forbear (omit) action is either to *leave* something *unchanged* or to *let* something *happen*'.[19]

Whenever a decision has been made not to prolong the life of a patient various courses of action have to be made. Is there to be a hastening of death ('killing') — a consequence produced either intentionally, or as a side effect through, for

example, the administration of analgesics to alleviate pain —
or is the patient to be given ordinary nursing care and
'allowed to die' or 'nature left to take its course'? Ramsey
(1970) describes the decision to withhold or withdraw therapy
as 'ceasing to do something that was begun in order to do
something that is better because it is now more fitting'.
Commenting on these questions Mr Richard Cook declared:

> 'Withholding treatment known very likely to succeed is
> *not* ethically different from terminating life (cf. not stop-
> ping a child seen to be about to run across a busy road).
> But risks of treatment and prospects of its success need to
> be assessed and a course of treatment should not be
> started unless it can be completed. Letting die (with
> accompanying love and care and attention to basic
> needs) is very different from accelerating or causing
> death by withholding normal entitlements (e.g. not feed-
> ing). We need to balance the *commandment* (not to kill)
> with *compassion*.'

To Professor Alan Emery there is ethically no difference:

> 'If the person withholding treatment has the ability and
> training to treat and therefore prevent death, then his
> withholding treatment is logically no different from
> actively terminating life. So to me there is little difference
> between these various acts.'

Dr Margaret White pointed out how important it is

> 'to distinguish between the act of omission which *causes*
> death (e.g. not operating on a duodenal atresia because
> the child has Down's syndrome), and where the act of
> omission applies to a second factor arising where some-
> one is already dying of something else in the near future.
> For example, there is no point in treating anencephalic
> babies for anything because they always die in a few days
> if not immediately after birth.'

Dr Jonathan Glover, as a philosopher, was inclined to think
that in principle there is no difference, and that it is a
distinction which ultimately is extraordinarily hard to defend
as being of any moral significance in itself:

'In many instances it's not absolutely clear what the boundary between killing and simply withholding treatment is. If we have someone on a respirator and then we switch it off, well, is that killing or is it merely withdrawing treatment — no longer taking positive steps? Where is the boundary? But that's not the central point. The central point is that in assessing the morality of two things people do or fail to do, there are two plausible candidates which make a moral difference. One is a difference of consequences. The other possible candidate is the difference in a person's intention. Now in many of the cases where there are two possible strategies for bringing about death there's the same consequence and the same intention in each case. . . . I find it extraordinarily hard to see why, in a case where the intention and the consequences are equivalent, we should attach any moral significance to what particular course of activity or non-activity happened to be adopted. That isn't to say of course there's never *any* place for the distinction between killing or failing to save life.'

He continued: 'It's much easier in law to prohibit a rather clearly defined class of action than a class of omission. For example, are we all murderers because we don't send money to Oxfam? Clearly the law could not enforce that kind of thing.

We've got to draw the line somewhere and we want, as it were, a clear-cut case with sharp boundaries rather than blurred boundaries. In some cases we may want to draw the line so that it coincides with the distinction between acts and omissions. The fact is that people find it much harder as doctors, say, to administer a lethal injection than to withhold treatment. Because of these factors in our psychology, which I don't think necessarily reflect values that are ultimately defensible, but are simply features of our responses, we may sometimes want to draw the line between acts and omissions but, in itself, apart from these side considerations, I can see no importance in that kind of distinction at all.'*

*Dr Jonathan Glover expands on these views in his book *Causing Death and Saving Lives*, Pelican, 1977.

Mr Michael Lockwood was not *quite* as convinced, perhaps, as Jonathan Glover that there is no ethical significance in this distinction:

> 'Broadly speaking, though, I am inclined to think that if you take pairs of cases in which the *only* distinguishing feature is that one involves an act where the other involves an omission, there will then be little if anything to choose between them, morally speaking. Suppose the pair of cases involve killing and letting die. If the intentions are the same and everything else is the same, then I'm inclined to think that the mere fact that, in the one case, death comes about because of something you positively do, whereas, in the other case, death comes about because of something you deliberately omit to do in order that death should result, cannot, at any rate, be of much moral significance.'

When I put the questions to Professor Ian Kennedy he thought that

> 'none of the people working in the field would be happy with the term "withholding treatment".'

A better way of analysing it, he felt, is to say

> 'there are certain circumstances when you change your treatment. You don't withhold in the sense that you neglect or abandon the patient.'

He also stressed it was important to define what 'treatment' really is, and that was by no means easy:

> 'For example, you have to ask yourself if feeding or giving fluids is treatment. There are some interesting arguments whether it may be or not. But what people would argue, who are engaged in terminal care, is that they don't withhold, they *change* their treatment. They change it from a treatment for the living, to a treatment for the dying. That means they may nurse, they may make comfortable; they change, wash, and if certain things happen, they respond to them. That is a form of treatment, a treatment of just keeping comfortable or reducing pain rather than acting vigorously. Ethically

one is entitled at some point to change the nature of one's treatment and treat for dying.'

Then, of course, the question is, 'When is that point?'.

'It's the same problem whether it be at the beginning or the end of life, and you have to work out what the criteria are. It may not apply to some neonates in the baby care unit, for a neonate may not be dying. The neonate may however be severely disabled. Then the question becomes whether you can encourage or permit it to die, if it doesn't respond in a certain way. If, on the other hand, it is a terminally ill baby, who by very definition may die sooner rather than later, the problem is one of caring for its dying from the outset. As regards the severely handicapped baby, you have to decide whether there is a point beyond which, or below which, to help them to hold on to life by whatever means you can, is morally unjustifiable.'

He thought that we have to work out what the thing the Americans call 'the bottom line' is; at which point the treatment is ethically uncalled for:

'It's easier in the context of the terminally ill, provided one is sure about the diagnosis, than as regards the severely handicapped newly-born, where the patient is not dying but has at the best the chance of a very poor life. With the terminally ill I have no problem. At some point they simply have to die. The difficulty with the neonate is that you are saying, the child is not dying, but you will in fact encourage it to die. I would set the threshold — the bottom line — very low. When you ask about killing or letting die, I would countenance it only in the severest cases of disability when there was no prospect of the child coming to any capacity to fulfil itself as a human being.'

As in this analysis no mention has been made of 'killing' or 'letting die', because the notion of changing one's treatment has been used, the question can be asked, 'Is it ever treatment to kill?', or if one does not use the word 'kill' shall we say 'hasten death', and here it is very difficult:

> 'I would have thought the better answer is to ask another question — "Is it really ever necessary to hasten death, so that in effect you really have to kill the patient?" I would have thought the answer is "very rarely". After all, the doctor already has the moral tool of the double effect theory, that is to say that although his primary intention is to relieve suffering, it may also be the case that death is also intended, in that it will predictably follow from the course of treatment adopted. But if it is intended as a secondary effect, this may be morally justified.'

Who Makes The Decisions?

Who has the onus to decide that life with a handicap, even a severe one, is not worth living? On what ethical principles can a choice be made?

> 'The choice is not between killing and keeping alive', explained Mr Richard Cook, 'but rather between aiming for rehabilitation on the one hand, and providing palliative treatment and care on the other. The latter may not prolong life but will make it worth living. The ethical principles include the sanctity of human life, with the necessity for special care and consideration for the weak and defenceless, and the relief of suffering.'

A most significant fact was noted by Dr Margaret White:

> 'The suicide rate is lower in those people who are born "handicapped" than in those not born handicapped, so the handicapped obviously consider their lives worth living.'

There were other physicians who considered that the choice is with the affected individual (not applicable in the foetus), the parents, and society:

> 'In practical terms', replied Dr M. A. C. Ridler, 'the choice lies with the parents, constrained by the ethical limits or accepted practices of society and the law. Society may pre-empt the parental choice if it is

genuinely and realistically prepared to accept full caring support for the affected individual, with a guarantee that the affected individual will be given maximum hope of achieving the potential for development and a full life.'

That adults may properly make their own decisions was the viewpoint of Professor Joseph Fletcher:

'Since pre-competent persons cannot make decisions in tragic cases their parents, family or guardians can and should. In that order of priority. Choice should be on the basis of conflicting *values* (the quality of life), not on the basis of a universal negative *rule* (the sanctity of life).'

Dr Graham Clayden was of the opinion that those

'with experience, who are able to predict to a degree the future implications of a handicap in a baby and have the experience/training tactfully to communicate this to distressed parents, and who can distil the basic feelings of the parents and guide their decision, should assist.'

Responding to the second part of the question, he expressed the view:

'The principle that "quality weighs heavier than quantity" in life and that suffering for an individual should be avoided provided the means to avoid suffering do not provoke suffering in other individuals, e.g. parents or attendants.'

At Great Ormond Street Hospital, Mr Herbert Eckstein emphasized the importance of assessing each patient and each individual at each particular moment in time:

'You have to consider the family as a whole. Obviously the child comes first, but I think there is a big difference if this is baby number four and the parents already have three healthy children— that's one problem. If this is the first baby and they've tried ten years to have one, and the chances of another pregnancy are remote, I think on an otherwise identical baby I would give a different verdict for that reason.'

What was the opinion of the philosophers? Dr Jonathan

Glover advised full co-operation between parents and doctor, with the final choice being left to the parents:

'It seems to me just as difficult a decision requiring no more, no less moral presumption to decide in some of the hard cases that a life is worth living as it is to decide that it isn't worth living. The person deciding has a great responsibility to them whatever way the decision goes. It's not true that simply letting nature take its course and making sure that the child stays alive is always morally an easier or less presumptuous a decision to take than a decision that the child might have a life which is not worth living, and that one should act accordingly. My own feeling is that what is needed is a lot of conversation between parents and medical advisers, because the parents of a seriously handicapped child usually don't know in advance very much about what the condition entails, and so it would be bad to suggest that they just discuss it on their own without any medical advice. But equally I feel uneasy about what is quite often the practice — that the final decision rests with the doctor, because the parents often have much more idea of what their particular family circumstances are like. It would be better if in most cases the final decision was at least predominantly with the parents. Now I realize that there are complications about this, because of course doctors can be prosecuted, and I certainly wouldn't suggest that doctors should be forced to take positive steps to kill a child. We wouldn't want to make them do that, and it would be morally wrong to do so. But I certainly think that where doctors are prepared to countenance either positive or negative euthanasia in the case of a severely handicapped child, then it is entirely appropriate that the parents should have the dominant say.'

Mr Michael Lockwood added some further relevant points:

'In my view the answer to the question, who should decide whether the child is to live or die, should depend, in part, on who is going to have to bear the burden of caring for the child if it lives. If the assumption is that if it lives the parents are going to be the ones looking after it, then it seems to me clear that they should have the dominant say. If, on the other hand, there is the option of the State caring for the child, in a way that would be acceptable to the parents, then it seems reasonable that the relevant agents of the State should have some say too.'

Another important point that needs to be made, he continued, was that

'the question rather implies that the only point at issue is whether the child's life is going to be worth living. But of course I might, as a parent, feel that the child's life probably would be worth living, in the sense that its life was likely to have some positive value, but that neverthe-less, it was unlikely to be sufficiently valuable to justify my sacrificing so much of my life in order to care for it. One has to balance whatever positive value the child's life may have in itself against the negative effects that the child may have on the lives of the parents, and the siblings if there are any. As I say, even if one decided that the child's life was worth living in itself, I don't think that would settle the question whether it ought to be allowed to live. There are these other considerations that have to be balanced against that.'

There is no denying that the family ought to have an important stake in the decision, for their whole life may be profoundly affected by what is to be decided. In their distress many find it difficult if not impossible to view the problem objectively. They will rely heavily on the judgement of the physician and his team. Dr Jack Insley outlined what nor-mally happens:

'Most parents when faced with the situation say, "Well you are the one who can make that sort of decision and we'll abide by what you say". Some will say, "Well, I accept your opinion and I would like to go home and talk about it". So you will have some who will accept the doctor's decision there and then, and others who will want to discuss it in much greater depth. There are religious families who will want to go and talk to their priest about it, and those in big family groups, especially the Asian families, may want to go and discuss it with their family and their relations. I think it's rather nice that they have someone else to talk to.'

They will naturally be ambivalent. In the majority of instances they want the baby to live, not die, yet the prospect of suffering and a lifelong responsibility for a handicapped child may initially overwhelm them. They cannot imagine at this stage what it will be like to raise a child with acute and serious physical and mental defects. Regardless of the outcome, the majority of parents feel guilty and need much compassionate support.

If the choice lies predominantly with the parents, are they competent to be decision-makers when they are in a state of shock? Whilst agreeing that parents would be involved in the decision, the physicians were not entirely happy about implicating them should they be in a highly emotional state. Yet delay may cause further emotional trauma. Professor A. E. H. Emery expressed the need for the utmost discretion:

> 'Care and tact is required in choosing the right moment, but certainly they (the parents) must be involved.'

The danger of any pressure being placed on the parents was raised by Mr Richard Cook:

> 'Parents are rarely in a position to understand or view matters objectively. To force them to make such decisions will almost inevitably lead to later feelings of guilt. "Have we killed a child who might have done better than we thought?" or "We are responsible for all his suffering because we kept him alive."
> The Revd G. Wenham in *Christian Graduate* of June 1982 wrote, "Parental unwillingness to care for their child no more justifies infanticide than a child's reluctance to care for an aged parent justifies euthanasia".'

The delicate skill and care needed by the doctor and all who are involved was emphasized by Dr Graham Clayden:

> 'The skill of those working with parents at these

moments should be to make a careful but rapid assessment of how the *particular individual* parents may cope. Whether they will continue to feel guilty or bitter about either being involved or not in any decisions, I think parents should be the main deciders, but the doctor should detect the underlying, often not yet uttered, decision and then feed back to the parents the decision as if from him, so the parents can face the suggested conclusion openly and discuss between them and the doctor. This puts a great responsibility on the doctor to know and combat his own prejudice and know how stressed parents react at different periods after the shock'.

How extremely difficult it often is for the doctor to adopt an objective role was indicated by Mr Herbert Eckstein:

'My impression has been that the vast majority of parents will either say, "You're the doctor, you know best. You decide whatever you think is right", or you are going to put the words into their mouths, unintentionally even, and they will come up with the decision you wanted. Very occasionally it's a baby I'm sure is worth treating, and the parents say, "No, on no account". Then, for once, I will try very hard to talk them out of that, and, on the whole, we have succeeded. More difficult is the situation where we feel the baby is best not treated yet the parents feel it must be treated at any price, by any means available and more or less insist on this.'

Further practical difficulties were outlined by Dr Iain Chalmers:

'The actual practicalities of engaging the parents in discussion at a time when real life and death decisions have to be taken are enormous. Even if one could engage in discussion with the parents, things would be happening the whole time which could determine a baby's mortality or survival. It's one thing to identify the right framework in which the decision should be taken and within which the problems should be addressed; but actually bridging the gap between a well considered framework and the

practicalities that face people on the ground, both
parents and doctors, is a very big issue which I don't
think has been adequately addressed. There is so very
little time — it's a question of whether you put a tube
down *now* into this tiny human being. After that it is a
cascade of further interventions to keep it alive unless the
decision is made to withdraw.'

To come to the practicalities, continued Dr Chalmers:

'Under the glaring lights of a hundred per cent hospital
confinement it is extremely difficult for any doctor to take
the sort of independent action that would be possible in
other circumstances. People behave defensively in these
circumstances, and the way they defend themselves is
usually to *do* things rather than *not* to do them. This
imposes constraints because the circumstances of child-
birth have changed.'

Both Dr Jonathan Glover and Professor William Silverman
introduced the interesting suggestion of discussion with
parents-to-be about handicapped babies and their personal
apprehensions and attitudes:

'It might be a good idea', propounded Jonathan Glover,
'to move over to a system where this question is raised at
an early stage of pregnancy — say in classes in hospitals,
where people can discuss the issue as an hypothetical
issue, rather than in moments of great distress and emotional pressure, so that some guidelines can be given in
advance to the doctors. There are obvious defects to this;
one is that it's hard to take hypothetical questions seriously; it is hard to think yourself fully into the position
imaginatively what it's really going to be like. Nevertheless I think there is something to be said for raising it;
that some preliminary guidelines are laid down in the
doctor's mind by the kinds of attitudes that are displayed
beforehand.'

The point made by Professor Silverman was that many, if not
most, parents have a fear of an untoward outcome but are
reluctant to mention or discuss this openly. They are even

reluctant to speak to each other, as husband and wife. One of the reasons why he felt rather strongly about such preparation was that as a physician he had seen

'malformed infants in the delivery room. All who are there — anaesthetist, obstetrician, paediatrician, nurses — have had many opportunities to review their own attitudes and preferences, except the parents who've not discussed it with one another. So, I argue, we need to explore ways and means of providing parents with an opportunity to consider their emotional and spiritual attitudes about unfavourable pregnancy outcome — in advance of the unlikely event. Some parents may not wish to raise such disturbing thoughts to consciousness, but for others who've been brooding about a dread possibility it might bring great relief. It's a delicate issue and should be approached gingerly. Parents should not be made to feel any pressure to discuss these difficult questions. I do argue, however, that the opportunity for review of attitudes during pregnancy should be made available — only then can we judge the extent to which some parents wish to prepare for an active role when it comes to deciding the fate of malformed offspring.'

Dr Silverman drew an interesting parallel with airline procedure:

'It's very much like the situation on getting on an aeroplane; you sit there and the stewardess says: "In the event of landing in the ocean here's how to put on a life jacket." Airlines fought the procedure saying, "Most flights are not going to crash. You are triggering fears in our happy passengers!" Its very much that kind of issue.'

Dr Margaret White saw no need for any life/death questions to be raised either ante or post-natal:

'Life or death questions should not be asked of parents at all at any time. A doctor's duty is to his patient — in this case the new born child. The doctor must do his best for his patient. If he can save the life of a child he must do so. If he can't there's no point in discussing it with the

> parents. This does not mean that operations which have little chance of success should be performed — just because they might possibly cause alleviation and will certainly cause the child distress.'

The doctor responsible for the care of the mother and child has to make a decision about what he thinks should be done, consulting colleagues if necessary, and discussing the problem with the entire team. In turn he has to report the situation to the family and be responsive to their wishes. It is the doctor, of course, who is in the best position to make a medical recommendation. He has to be aware that his decision can be easily and unconsciously swayed by feelings of sympathy and prejudice which may be irrelevant to the main issue at hand. He has to guard against his emotions overriding his logic.

Some people are of the opinion that committees with medical, legal and theological representatives should be responsible for review in certain intricate cases involving limitation of intervention, but the majority of doctors view such groups as 'clumsy instruments' for vital decision-making. Not only are there the practical problems of convening a group of this kind at short notice during times of crises, but there is the additional difficulty of informing them of all the medical and social complexities of a clinical situation. Franz J. Ingelfinger (1973) while agreeing that society, ethics, institutional attitudes and committees may well provide the broad guidelines, asserts that the onus of decision-making must ultimately fall on the doctor who is caring for the child.[20] This was a view shared by many other physicians.[21] Dr Graham Clayden considered that

> 'as these decisions are based on so many other variables, many of which are impossible to define, measure or weigh, a committee decision would be crude at best.'

Dr Janet Goodall was equally firmly convinced that

> 'decision by committee could be disastrous and decision by a court insensitive. Parents and child must be known as individuals to those who cast the votes.'

No ethical distinction was seen by Dr Thomas Mawdsley

between the handicapped and their peers, so it followed that

> 'the decisions regarding treatment are medical and parental, but certainly not for committees.'

A number of doctors thought it helpful for parents to discuss such decisions with professional advisers, social workers and priests.

Duff and Campbell (1973) are of the opinion that if families are given information and answers to their questions in words they understand, the problems of their children as well as the expected benefits and limits of any proposed care can be understood clearly in all instances.[22] It is the experience of many paediatricians that parents when greatly stressed and emotionally upset are still capable of sharing difficult decisions and benefit by so doing.

There are those who feel that as these issues involved are more moral than medical and scientific, doctors and parents are not always qualified to make these life-death decisions.[23] They advocate that it is a task of a community much broader than the medical community, for the ultimate decisions about life and death are not simply medical decisions as Professor Ian Kennedy made plain in his Reith Lectures of 1981.

As Peter Baelz, Dean of Durham, sensitively put it:

> 'It's easy to talk when you are not involved. When you are involved, then (1) you have to act, (2) you are acutely sensitive to other people involved. But I think there's a lot to be said for working out your principles in a relatively cool situation when you are not simply moved by emotion. The two should go together. There is a time for thinking, and a time for testing your thoughts by the situation you find yourself in. We cannot simply leave things to the doctors. The doctors cannot simply leave the decision to parents, who need help and support when they are suddenly told they have an abnormal baby. Some clinical decisions have moral elements built into them, because they are concerned in part with what kind of life is worth living and that is not just a clinical question.'

Where there are conflicting viewpoints between paediatri-

cians and parents the former will normally either accept the
wishes and decisions of the latter, or refer the infant to the care
of a colleague who may be more in sympathy with the parental beliefs and opinions.[24] Some aspects of this problem were
explained to me by Professor William Silverman as we sat
together in Helen House, Oxford:*

> 'In my own interviewing of parents of newly-blinded
> children they repeatedly told me: "I was quite unable to
> tell the doctors what I wanted". Parents felt powerless to
> express what they wanted in the circumstances.' Dr
> Silverman continued, 'As a physician, I have been con-
> vinced that I don't know what they want and when I ask
> them in the setting of the hospital, I control the answer.
> The very words I use control the answer. When I ask
> them questions the answers are different from those that
> those same parents give to their friends or to their minis-
> ter. I'd like to measure how different the answer would
> be if I changed the enquirer, or changed the setting from
> hospital to home. If we find the frequency of the mis-
> match to be significant, that would seem a good reason
> for providing an alternative.'

Distressed families should never be allowed to feel that
they alone are left to make major and crucial decisions, and
that everything depends on them. They have a tendency to
make up their minds contrary to their real beliefs, because
they think that their relatives, friends, church, or doctor will
not approve; feelings of guilt may be aroused if they later
come to the conclusion they have made the 'wrong decision'.
No doctor should be 'a mere technician' who presents the
facts, steps back, waits for the parents to make their decision, and then performs the medical or surgical service
requested by them. It is important that the final decision is
made in such a way as to avoid placing an impossible
burden on them. The *Handbook of Medical Ethics* (BMA,

---

* Helen House, 37 Leopold Street, Oxford, OX4 1QT, is a hospice which
  gives day to day love and care to gravely ill children and supports their
  families. It was founded in 1982 by Mother Frances Dominica, Superior
  General of the Anglican Society of All Saints, Oxford.

1981) suggests that 'for an infant the parents must ultimately decide' with 'the responsible physician (helping) the parents to understand the choices' (p. 32). Decisions are best made together in an atmosphere of full disclosure, of support for the family and above all else, of loving and understanding concern for each newborn.

> 'Parents expect cure, and hope for miracles', explained Dr Ralph Evans. 'The truth is that cure is impossible, and miracles occur but rarely. It is imperative that nothing be done to suggest to the parents that non-treatment is equated with "non-caring". The non-treated child and his parents probably require *more* sympathetic care and help than the treated.'

Impact on the Family

When a severely handicapped infant is born the family normally experience two distinct emotional grief reactions as they confront 'the terror of death in the sublime moments of birth'. There is the loss of the 'perfect' baby that was expected, and the sudden birth of a rather feared threatening defective infant. One mother described her feelings as those of 'total inadequacy, total failure, because deep down you feel that your first job is that your child should survive and you have failed'. Another parent graphically stated: 'It is like being tossed around in a stormy sea. There are no anchors, no certainties about anything at all. Your life, for the moment, has been shattered'. The news should always be broken to the two parents together at an early stage (some paediatricians say not later than the second day). Dr Hugh Jolly explained:

> 'You should never tell parents and discuss these things with parents separately. Yet there are still people who say, "Tell father first and then leave him to tell mother." I'm sure that father and mother have got to be told together. In the telling I've been very influenced by parents who have emphasized, "Please tell your staff not to start the conversation with, 'I've got bad news', or something like that. We want the facts whether its bad news or not. It's our job not yours, so please give us the facts".'

The majority of parents seem to resent any delay in hearing what has happened.

It is not possible to make a comprehensive assessment of the effects of having a severely handicapped child born into the family, for the capacity for coping with the child will vary. There will be some parents who reveal quite unsuspected courage whilst others seem quite unable to cope. So much depends upon the circumstances and characteristics of the parents. Several studies have been undertaken of the initial reactions of parents. Hare *et al.* (1966) interviewed parents of 120 infants with spina bifida within three days of birth and later, and showed how fathers expressed more distress than mothers when the news was broken, but mothers found it difficult to 'take in' the situation so soon after delivery.[25] The effect of the baby's handicap and/or death often lasts longer with the father than the mother, and the care and advice given to the mother should not neglect the father.

Reactions to the birth of a handicapped child are somewhat similar to the stages of grief in the more normal settings of death and dying. There is mourning for the child mother had planned to produce. To grief there may be added feelings of shame, bewilderment, as well as a primitive sense of being punished for wrong-doing. Feelings of anger will often be much in evidence. Hostility may be projected on God, the doctors or staff in charge. How could God be so cruel? Why did not the doctor do 'this' or 'that'? There will be disbelief: 'I can't believe its true!' 'There's been a mix-up.' 'It's all a mistake.' 'Why has it happened to me?' 'Will it happen again?' As another mother put it: 'It didn't seem fair; it didn't seem right at all. All I wanted to do was to cuddle him. I kept on thinking it was a dream.'

Much of the reaction will depend on how the news is broken to the parents. They seem to remember very little about the interview with the doctor other than the *way* in which they were told — 'he was very kind', 'he was obviously upset himself'. Not only must there be time for parents to assimilate the facts but also for the medical team to gain more information about the family itself. Their 'mourning' is somewhat relieved if something is being done for the child such as a surgical operation. A number of those parents who had refused surgery for their child in the initial stages were prone to express how guilty they felt when they realized their baby was not going to die immediately.[26]

Where parents anticipate terminal care of their infant they will probably commence their grief before the actual death takes place. Many of them are normally helped by being involved, whenever it might be possible, in the management of their baby — to help cuddle, wash, feed, give comfort and love. Any attempt to suppress, control or postpone acute grief responses by prescribing tranquillizers or anti-depressant drugs too readily will only serve to prolong the eventual process of grieving.

Parents gain much comfort from the knowledge that everything that can be done is being done, and that, where it is so, the condition of the infant is in no way their fault and will not recur in subsequent pregnancies. If the baby is referred to by his christian name, and touched and handled as befits his condition as one who still has dignity and value, no matter how severely handicapped he may be, this has a profound impression on the parents. They are greatly helped by having physical contact or at least visual contact with their child. Very few mothers ever regret seeing a handicapped baby, for it seems to save them from 'a mysterious frightening secret'. This was the opinion of Dr Jolly:

> 'If you don't show a grossly handicapped child then one reaction of parents is, "It's so bad the doctor can't even show it to me!". I think that the imagined "monster" is always worse.'

Dr Jack Insley described the procedures adopted in his Infant Development Unit:

> 'What we like to do is to remove all the tubes and everything so that the baby looks human. We dress him and take him to the mother who would be in a private room in the unit, and let the baby die in mother's arms and father's arms too if he's there. This seems highly beneficial in the long term because they have been there at the end, and perhaps it's easier to accept. We always offer them the opportunity of seeing the child. Then they

say quite often, "Well, what a lovely face", and so on. I think doctors have underestimated over the years human emotion and response, and probably still do.'

An almost identical viewpoint was expressed by Dr Jolly:

'If you've got a very small premature baby in an intensive care unit, and it is going to die, it will probably die with lots of machinery all on it, respirator and so on. The parents, other than touching the baby through the ports, will never have held their baby. Now not only should they hold the baby, but — and this is a very important point — they should be offered to dress the baby. This is the first real caring and human thing they've been able to do to their baby. Since we initiated this it's made a tremendous difference.'

He went on to describe what is actually done:

'Baby must be taken out of the incubator and all the machinery taken off. The parents then have the chance of holding their baby, who looks like a real baby instead of a "machine-man", where everything is covered with electrodes, monitors, and respirators. Then baby is photographed with them.'

The value and help of having a photograph taken was reiterated by the remarks of some of the mothers. 'I value the pictures of S. around the house', said one mother. 'I have a feeling that because of the pictures he is still with us.' Another explained, 'We need something to show we have had a baby — to dispel the sense of having merely experienced a bad dream.'

One mother records her great distress at not being allowed to see her hydrocephalic baby: 'They never asked me if I'd like to see the baby. I woke up in the evening and nobody said a word about the baby, what sex it was or what it weighed. If only I'd got a lock of hair to prove I had something. They could have wrapped him up so I could see, covered the back of his head or something. When I left that hospital, I was left with *nothing*.' Another, in contrast, who was shown her dead baby by the nurse who commented how beautiful he was, reflects: 'He was beautiful . . . I can picture him now. He had little rosy cheeks. Seeing him was an amazing good thing to have done.' She was given opportunity to say 'hello' to her dead baby, which made her the more able to say 'goodbye'.[27] Dr Hugh Jolly stated that he always finds, in talking to mothers whose baby has been delivered dead, that they have a name for the baby:

> 'I don't say: "Did the baby have a name?" I merely say: "What was the baby's name?" — they always have one.'

A baby should never be referred to as 'the spina bifida', 'the Down's syndrome', or the unforgivable 'it'.

A parent's grief response to the birth of a handicapped infant is of course highly individualized and may depend more on the love, understanding and compassion of those who are involved in their care than any other single factor.[28] After-care of the parents is extremely important and a challenge to the caring and supportive community and congregation. They must not be left to feel abandoned, ostracized, with an unmanageable burden on their hands. Such community support from friends and neighbours is often difficult to arrange and some families seem shut in their own homes. In a Newcastle spina bifida study by Walker *et al.* (1971) only twenty-six per cent of families received any help from neighbours and many parents found the curiosity of strangers disconcerting. Mitchell (1973) comments that perhaps the most hurtful thing is the feeling of rejection by friends and neighbours. 'Such remarks as "more and more friends stopped visiting us and always put me off if I suggested visiting them", and "people are very good at sympathizing with you but when it comes to giving practical help, they don't want to know you", bear eloquent testimony to the indifference and even callousness shown by many people towards handicapped children and their families.'[29]

Alongside feelings of guilt there may be an awareness of self-blame, social stigma, feelings of inadequacy, or inferiority, and searching questionings. Often parents seem most anxious to discover the cause for the abnormalities of the baby and look for reasons within the respective families. Zachary (1968) comments that 'the wife's knowledge about the husband's ancestors is only equalled by that of the husband's knowledge of the wife's ancestors'.[30] It is difficult for them to tolerate a state of having *no* satisfactory reason why their baby has been born handicapped or abnormal.

For those who are unable to cope with the future care of a handicapped child or have rejected it outright, and are reluctant for the baby to be placed in an institution, there may possibly be an opportunity for the infant to be adopted, rather than letting him die. Adoption obviously is extremely difficult, but there are encouraging signs that there are families who are ready to care for and bring up a handicapped baby. The organization, "Parents for Children", states that 'in the last five years this agency alone has placed twenty-two mentally handicapped and twelve physically handicapped children for adoption' (*The Times*, 25 August 1981). Adoption of handicapped children seems to becoming more common.

Professor William Silverman expressed his concern about the conditions under which some handicapped and extremely premature neonates die. He advocated that the problems of providing a humane, natural death for these infants might be eased were they nursed somewhere other than in an intensive care unit. As hospices have been founded to allow adults to die in peace and dignity away from an atmosphere of therapeutic intervention, so infants might be transferred to a comparable environment. He regarded Helen House, Oxford, where our discussion took place, as ideally suited to the needs of such an evaluation. In such a setting both parents and child would have the necessary emotional and spiritual support to allow the child to die under loving and caring conditions:

> 'The physical setting of a modern intensive care unit, with its panoply of rescue machinery, blares out the non-verbal message of life prolongation — that message drowns out any murmurings concerning the idea of "natural death", and medical rescuers see anything less than life support as non-treatment. The concept of least-not-cruelty is foreign to those obsessed by a rescue fantasy.'

He felt strongly that medicine should openly admit that it cannot be expected to deal with the problem of humane natural death for malformed and extremely premature neonates once decisions had been made.

Personhood

In order to justify some of the life-death decisions which have to be made in the circumstances described, it is important to attempt to define what a 'meaningful' life really is. What does it mean to be a 'person'? Is there such a thing as 'a life not worth living'? Fletcher (1979) states that, 'In biomedical ethics writers constantly say that we need to explicate human-ness or humaneness, what it means to be a truly human being, but they never follow their admissions of the need with an actual inventory or profile, no matter how tentatively offered. Yet this is what must be done, or at least attempted.' He suggests that humanhood or personhood is conferred by other humans upon the fulfilment of certain qualitative and quan-titative indicators, and unless a human being possesses these capacities he cannot be counted as a person. He proposes fifteen positive propositions or 'indicators': minimum intelli-gence, self-awareness, self-control, a sense of time, a sense of futurity, a sense of the past, the capacity to relate to others, concern for others, communication, control of existence, curiosity, change and changeability, balance of rationality and feeling, idiosyncrasy, neocortical function.[31]

The most important medical criterion according to Duff and Campbell (1979) is the degree of abnormality, disease or damage to the central nervous system, especially the brain. If there is little or no prospect of brain function sufficient to allow a personal life of meaning and quality, or no potential for development in harmony with Fletcher's 'indicators of humanhood', they see non-treatment as the prudent course of action.[32] Some, like McCormick (1974), are of the opinion that human life is not an absolute good, but is relative to the other goods for whose attainment it is the necessary condition. He sees the essence of a meaningful life as an ability to form relationships. In an attempt to find a guideline which may help in decisions about sustaining the lives of grossly deformed and deprived infants, he feels that, if the potential for human relationships is simply non-existent or would be utterly submerged and undeveloped in the mere struggle to survive, that life has achieved its potential. The guidelines are not seen to be a detailed rule that pre-empts decisions, and mistakes may be made; but allowing some infants to die does not imply that 'some lives are valuable, others are not', or that 'there is such a thing as a life not worth living', for every life, regardless of age or condition, is of incalculable worth.[33]

Paul Ramsey (1978) sees both the fetus and the new born infant as possessing humanhood of irreducible dignity as a free gift of God, and considers that decisions to treat or not to treat should be the same for the normal and the abnormal alike.[34]

A recent Report (1980) of the Anglican Church of Canada Task Force on Human Life,[35] in its interim statement to the 1977 session of the 28th General Synod of the Church of Canada, stated quite categorically concerning severely handicapped infants that 'our senses and emotions lead us into the grave mistake of treating human-looking shapes as if they were human, although they lack the least vestige of human behaviour or intellect. In fact the only way to treat such defective infants humanely is not to treat them as human'. After a controversy over this statement (*New York Times*, 28 July 1977) the viewpoint was considerably modified in the revised draft of the Report to read: 'It cannot be asserted too strongly that, so long as such individuals might attain a minimal degree of self-determination or can engage in some social interaction, they are indeed persons, even though they lack the potential to reach the level of personal development open to those of us who are not so afflicted. . . . Having accepted the argument that retarded infants are indeed possessed of personhood, one is morally bound to afford them the necessary surgical aid and to all continued life' (p. 41).

The doctors, philosophers and ethicists with whom I discussed the definition of 'personhood' saw intercommunication and relationship to be among its essential elements. Self-awareness and communication formed part of Dr Graham Clayden's definition:

> 'A physical organism reaches a "person" when he or she can communicate with others or be aware of himself/herself. This communication may be extremely difficult, e.g. severe cerebral palsy. Our materialistic view of life and intelligence may make us blind to some essence of "personhood" in a severely handicapped child, however

an open minded attendant may "feel" or "know" the difference at some levels of severe handicap.'

Dr Jonathan Glover emphasized the gradual evolvement of personhood and defined it in a broad spectrum:

'The concept of personhood isn't a simple concept and the question, "when does a fetus or baby become a person?" is something more like, "when does middle age begin?" than like the question, "when did the light get switched on in such and such a room?" I think that what inclines us to say that somebody is a person is a whole cluster of different things — it's being conscious, having a certain range of conceptual abilities to be able to understand certain things: it's having an emotional life, relationships with other people. It's a whole range of different things which may not have a moment of onset but may gradually evolve with the developing nervous system at various stages of pregnancy.'

A further point was added by Mr Michael Lockwood — that of self-awareness:

'Something else that I think is of considerable moral significance is this business of having a conception of oneself, as a being with a past and a future, a certain kind of self-reflective consciousness. It seems to me that the ability to have a conception of oneself, in this sense, and to form plans for one's life and so on, is a very large element in what makes the particular biological organism that we call a person especially ethically significant.'

To Dr Peter Singer also 'personhood' is to be defined as:

'The capacity for self-awareness — that is, the ability to see oneself as an independent entity with a past and a future.'

Mr Richard Cook, as a paediatrician, saw it as

'a status conferred, not one earned by realizing an arbitrary standard of intelligence or emotional response. Every child (foetus or born) must be considered to have the potential of humanity of "personhood". This will be

very obvious to most parents if they are involved in the
care of their infant — however weak or handicapped he
may seem to be.'

The very ambiguity of the term 'person' can lead to much
confusion and one has to define clearly one's terminology in
argument and debate. The word itself can be used in quite
different terms and senses, and Ian Kennedy was rightly
insistent about the importance of defining terms:

> 'If you take the view that "person" means having those
> qualities and attributes which a human being ordinarily
> would have, then anything that doesn't have those is not
> a person. It would then follow that you have built a
> rather dangerous definition of a person because you have
> a problem, for example, with neonates. They do not have
> certain capacities which human beings ordinarily have.
> You may have a problem with the unconscious. Senti-
> ence may be a criterion of being a person, yet it is only a
> criterion if you have told me what you want to use the
> word "person" for. For example, it would be a very
> dangerous criterion if you wanted to use the word "per-
> son" as indicating that which is owed respect, implying
> that when it is not a person it is not owed respect,
> because I would ask you, "All right, what would I do
> with my severely comatose patient?" It would depend on
> what sentience meant; whether it meant being aware of
> and interacting with the environment or merely respon-
> sive to painful stimuli. I would prefer as the criterion of
> being a person, being owed respect as a human being,
> the criterion of *capacity* to interact and demonstrate senti-
> ence. That would mean that if they have the capacity, as
> distinct from the actuality or not, at the present time, of
> using it, then you can still regard them as persons.'

The various attempts which have been made to define 'personhood' were summed up for me by Professor Joseph
Fletcher. He reiterated them as follows:

> '(1) just being alive, (2) being self-aware, (3) being
> aware of others.' He defended the view that 'it is best
> defined with cortical or cerebral function — this view (4)

making cerebral function the cardinal or essential function. It presupposes the other definitions (2) and (3). The only real antithesis is between (1) and (4).'

Any attempt at a rigid or dogmatic definition of 'personhood' is to be shunned, for decisions must always be reached and worked through individually with love and concern for each unique person. The christian understanding of human nature is expressed in the concept that man was created in the 'image' and 'likeness' of God ('God created man in his own image; in the image of God he created him; male and female he created them.' Gen. 1.27, NEB). Man is thus able to know and to love God, and to establish a personal relationship with him. We develop personhood in relation to other persons and ultimately in relationship to God. As Canon Gordon Dunstan expresses it, God 'created man in his own image, that is, with a potential for an identity capable of awareness of God, capable of a freely-willed response to the awakening or call of God, and therefore capable of a consequent likeness with God, of being stamped with his mark, his character, his image.' (*The Artifice of Ethics*, ibid p. 70)

The sanctity of life, the dignity and worth of each individual person, is not an achievement or an attribute conferred on him by others, but rather an endowment, a gift of God himself. Because of man's relationship to God humanity holds an unique place within his total creation.

It is inevitable, such is the diversity of opinions not only among physicians themselves but also between philosophers and ethicists, that the definition of personhood will become an ongoing debate. It is to be hoped that it will be one in which the Church will have a constructive contribution to make, for it is an issue in which the whole nature of man and his relation to God is involved.

Conclusions
As is evident, these issues raise the most agonizing, complex and sensitive moral problems, and discussions and debates are not exactly helped by emotional slogans or rigid dogmas. 'Untidy problems do not have tidy solutions' (Habgood 1980), and to these well nigh impossible situations there seem

no ready-made solutions. An honest appraisal of the situation
was given by one physician:

> 'Are we really judges of the quality of life? How biased
> each one of us can be in deciding what we think is the
> quality of life. I do not think we can be that judge. For
> those who think they can, my next question would be,
> how far do we have the right to go along with the
> decision we have made? That is an impossible question
> to answer. When can one decide that the quality of life
> could be so bad that we have the right not to take any
> measures to prolong it?'

The major issue at stake is respect for human life. All
human life is sacred. Every so-called 'imperfect' or 'handicapped' child, no matter how severe the disability, is still a
human being, a child of God. Medical or surgical techniques
should not be allowed to triumph over reason. What can be
done is not necessarily what should be done. In some instances it would seem that the best treatment is no treatment.
To preserve life at all costs, as if existence were the main or
only end to be achieved, is not always morally legitimate. On
the other hand intentionally to neglect or kill is to be
condemned.[36] A recent editorial in the *British Medical Journal*
warned that 'we must beware of that slippery slope that would
lead to the nonchalant taking of lives found to be substandard,
inconvenient, or expensive; but the "existence at-all-costs"
view points to a terrain no less treacherous. Letting nature
take it course in certain circumstances is to acknowledge that
there might sometimes be a right not to live — but we badly
need to clear our confusions about what these circumstances
are.'[37]

What constitutes an 'acceptable' quality of life? Such a
question raises other formidable problems as Dr Margaret
White was quick to point out:

> 'Acceptable to whom? The Jews were unacceptable to
> Hitler and the Aborigines to the early Australian settlers!
> There is no evidence that the severely mentally hand-
> icapped who live permanently in institutions are not
> happy. Thalidomide children do not commit suicide, but
> students (especially in Sweden) have a very high suicide
> rate.'

Dr White went on to relate how

> 'a film star (Liv Ullman) who was working temporarily
> for UNICEF, visited an African village after a drought.
> Outside a straw hut were eight smiling children. She
> asked her interpreter why they were smiling when they
> were so poor and had such a large family and such a
> filthy hut to live in. The interpreter replied: "They are all
> illiterate and therefore they cannot read the *New York
> Times*, and so they do not know that they are poor and
> without such necessities of life as coca-cola and televi-
> sion. They are smiling because they are a happy family."
> Our happiness depends almost entirely upon the quality
> of our personal relationships with other human beings.
> Those who have a poor quality of life in my experience
> are those who either through their own selfishness or
> misfortune have no close human contacts and are miser-
> ably lonely.'

Mr Richard Cook commented:

> 'Whatever its quality, there is a sense in which life has to
> be "accepted". We all have handicaps. There is no such
> thing as a perfect human being.'

The fact that most handicapped individuals learn to accept
their quality of life was endorsed by Professor Eugene
Diamond:

> 'Even severely handicapped children have been
> demonstrated to value their lives. Acceptance of a certain
> level of quality of life is in the eye of the beholder.
> Rejection of a certain quality of life may have more to do
> with its impact on relatives or the society at large.'

What had the philosophers to say here? Dr Jonathan Glover
confessed it was a most difficult question:

> 'The only way I can think about this is simply to do the
> sort of experiments philosophers have proposed, which
> have notorious inadequacy, such as to ask, "If I knew
> that I was going to have that sort of life or could die,
> which would I prefer to do?" Obviously it is extremely
> difficult and you will find different people giving different

answers to the thought experiments about the same sort
of condition. I think that is the nearest one can get.'

He thought that there was a lot to be said for giving particular
weight to consulting people about this — those who have
quite a lot of experience, either as parents or siblings or
doctors:

> 'But I think the fundamental question for each person is:
> "Do I think on balance this is the sort of life I myself
> would find worth living?" That is only the framework of
> the answer to one aspect of the question. I agree with the
> distinction that Michael drew earlier (see p.131) between
> the sort of case where we might want to say the child's
> life is worth living from his own point of view, but it's
> simply not worth it in terms of the wreck that is going to
> be made of the family life. Everything depends upon
> particular circumstances. Some families are enriched by
> this kind of experience; for many other families I'm quite
> sure it's a disaster. What one needs to do, I think, is to
> take into account both these points of view. In fact the
> test I have suggested, which is highly inadequate, is only
> part of the answer to one of these two questions.'

Some of the difficulties were reiterated by Gill Lockwood, a
clinical medical student:

> 'I've had it put to me, in something that sounds suspi-
> ciously like an argument that treats the child merely as a
> means rather than an end, that the Down's syndrome
> infant in a family so enriches the life of the family that
> what life may be like for the child becomes secondary to
> the effect of that child's life on the family. Sometimes that
> is a disaster; but sometimes it does appear to draw the
> family together and provide a focus for family harmony
> which enriches that family's life. But again, for an out-
> sider, even a doctor, to decide which situation is going to
> occur, at the point when a decision has to be made
> whether to provide or deny resuscitation, is clearly
> impossible.'

Unfortunately we live in an age when man is valued for what

he can do rather than for who he is; when life is seen as the ultimate good and death as the ultimate evil. It was heartening to be reminded by Dr Janet Goodall:

> 'Life is good, but death can also be good. There comes a time to let go. In both living and dying, we should offer help to the patient and hope to the parents, even if our shared hope is that the child's life will have been both bearable and memorable. The measure of life's value is not made in years. Even a brief life can be seen to have had purpose and influence.'

Professor R. S. Duff admirably summed up for me what is at stake:

> 'We live in an age of unprecedented scientific achievement. This gives us great powers and rich benefits. But in medicine as in defence we have terrible difficulties deciding how to use these new powers because we live in an age of moral darkness. In an enlightened age, this debate would be absurd, a step towards darkness. In this age of darkness, we must scrutinize the absurd in search of light.'

The author wishes to acknowledge his gratitude to Hugh Jolly, Late Department of Paediatrics, Charing Cross Hospital, London, for commenting upon and reading through the original draft of this chapter for medical accuracy.

5

Human Fertilization and Embryology

The majority of couples are able to plan their family on the assumption they are in complete control of their own fertility, but unfortunately there are still many who experience some difficulty in conceiving that planned child, for the problem of infertility affects about ten per cent of all partners. It is estimated that in forty per cent of instances the problem lies with the woman, forty per cent with the man, and twenty per cent with both husband and wife.

The Problem

A number of infertility cases are due to ovulatory disorders, others to blocked or damaged tubes as a result of infection. In male infertility many have few or no spermatozoa or there are deficiencies in the seminal fluid. The demand for treatment for infertility therefore is great. In recent years there have been considerable advances, and it is now estimated that approximately fifty per cent of couples seeking treatment eventually achieve a child of their own. Surgery, drugs and other therapies are continuously improving, and are offering more hope to sub-fertile couples, many of whom are deeply distressed and disturbed by their condition, for the problem of human infertility causes much anxiety, anguish, marital problems, and sometimes depression with suicidal tendencies.

Those who work with infertile couples acknowledge that there is a great deal of emotional stress imposed on some couples by the fact of their infertility. There are protracted periods of waiting, expecting a pregnancy and disappointment when the pregnancy does not come; discovering after a long tedious series of medical examinations, which are often unpleasant, that there is something wrong with one or other of the partners. Many see infertility as a challenge to their personality. As one partner put it: 'The trouble with infertility is that it's not just a physical condition — it's a social disease that needs medical treatment. Not only are couples afraid of coming forward to talk — they are also shy of talking to each other. It's the old fear of a man not being quite a man, a woman not quite a woman.'

In the past it has been possible for an infertile couple to adopt a child but there is at present an acute shortage of children for adoption. Access to effective contraceptives, freer availability of sterilizations, and increasing use of legal abortion have recently reduced the number of unplanned babies. Unmarried mothers are also more ready to keep their children. Figures published by the Office of Population Censuses and Surveys (1983) show a dramatic fall in the number of adoptions between 1974 and 1981 — from 22,000 children adopted in 1974 (figures for England and Wales) to just 9,000 in 1981. The scarcity of babies available seems to rule out the possibility of adoption for couples who are infertile because of the 'sterility' of the husband. There are, however, further options available to them.

AIH and AID

AIH (artificial insemination by the husband) is usually sought when the wife does not conceive after regular sexual intercourse, and the physician has diagnosed male infertility. Such infertility may be caused by impotence, anatomical defects of the urethra, physical disability or some defect or weakness in the quality of the sperm. Chances of pregnancy seem to be increased by concentrating the husband's semen or by inserting it directly into the uterus. AIH is now rather infrequently used, for AID (artificial insemination by donor) is simpler and considered more successful in securing a woman's pregnancy.

AID is used when the husband has been found to be infertile or to have significantly reduced fertility — a condition which could affect about 14,000 couples a year. This procedure has been practised in Britain for more than forty years, and is used not only for infertility problems but also where there is a risk of some serious hereditary genetic defect (for example, Huntington's chorea) being transmitted from the affected father to his children.

The actual process is extremely simple. Semen produced by masturbation is collected from an anonymous donor and is either used fresh or is frozen as quickly as possible and stored until it is used. (The proportion of successful inseminations is higher with fresh semen.) A fine syringe or catheter deposits the semen either into the upper portion of the vagina or directly into the woman's cervical canal. This takes place at the time of ovulation. Each potential recipient is required to keep accurate menstrual records and assessments are made of the likely timing of ovulation. Owing to the unpredictability of the exact timing two or more inseminations are often necessary at each cycle. The procedure is entirely painless and takes about twenty minutes. The ultimate success rate may be as high as seventy-five per cent (i.e. not seventy-five per cent success per ovulatory cycle).

Ideally both husband and wife will share in the desire to have a child, and in a mutually stable relationship freely and openly discuss their feelings about their infertility problem. Their motives for having children will, it is to be hoped, be based on mature judgement, and not simply on pressure from parents or in-laws. It is beneficial if they have together worked out some of the legal, social and moral issues with their general practitioner and/or priest. The majority of AID practitioners are very careful to leave the final decision to the couple concerned. Goldenberg and White (1977) report that in their practice they 'strongly believe that once provided with adequate information and counselling, each couple has the right to make their own choice. If the couple chooses AID we try only to determine if they are relatively comfortable with their decision, to discuss beforehand some of the possible conflicts they may have and then to proceed as they desire.'

Those AID practitioners who have published details of their work outline some of the various criteria used in the selection of couples. Some of the suggested criteria are as follows:

> Only strongly motivated couples are considered.
> The husband must be sterile, or subfertile, or possess rhesus incompatibility or adverse genetic factors.
> The wife must be free from hereditary disease and able to care for the child.

The wife must be mentally and physically able to care for the child.

There should be no deeply ingrained fears or prejudices about the practice.

There must be a mutual understanding between the husband and wife and an apparent potential mutual understanding between the mother and child and between the husband and child.

The family environment must be 'good'.

The couple must be 'childworthy'.

The life expectancy of both husband and wife should be reasonable.

The desire for a child should not be merely a response to peer or parental pressure.

The couple must be able to give the child suitable intellectual chances in life.[1]

In the past decade requests for AID have increased as the availability of babies for adoption becomes increasingly more difficult. It is now available on the National Health Service in certain parts of the country, and also in many private clinics. For many AID has distinct advantages over adoption which is seen as more impersonal, and there is often a stronger desire to 'bear' a child than to 'rear' one. An AID child is seen as 'our child', for mother carries it through all the problems and pleasures of nine months of pregnancy.

Sperm Banks

When stored in liquid nitrogen at very low temperatures sperm can maintain its viability indefinitely. Consequently sperm from numerous donors can, in this way, be maintained with the building up of sperm banks. Although medical research with frozen semen has been carried out for over twenty years, human sperm banks have only existed as a service in UK since 1970. Not only can sperm now be kept but also coded according to donor characteristics, so that a choice of donor sperm is available enabling the closest possible match in physical and mental characteristics between the donor and the husband. Already in the USA sperm banking is a lively business, spurred on by the rapidly increasing number of vasectomies (the cutting of the vas deferens tubes leading from the testicles to ensure sterility). In Britain the first such centre for human sperm was set up in Exeter some fifteen years ago, and other centres have recently been established. It is psychologically important that there be appropriate matching, and it is crucial that there be an avoidance of hereditary disease especially if the donor's semen be used repeatedly and anonymously.

With sperm banks now a reality, the selection of donors seems an awesome responsibility. A recent news item (*The Times*, 17 February, 1982) reported that an American company was offering frozen human sperm to European doctors by mail order. The late distinguished geneticist, H. J. Muller, of Indiana University, USA, proposed sperm banks with material derived from persons of outstanding gifts, intelligence, moral fibre and physical fitness. Such an idea, he propounded, would effect a great advance in human brotherhood, intelligence and bodily vigour. In 1979 the controversial sperm bank in Escondido, California, The Depository for Germinal Choice, announced it would accept only the sperm of Nobel prizewinners. Mr Robert Graham, an optometrist, the founder of the bank, states that he wants to think in terms of a few more creative, intelligent people who otherwise would not be born. At least five Nobel prizewinners are reported to have contributed to the sperm bank. There is, however, no guarantee that a child conceived from the sperm of a highly intelligent donor would be of similar intelligence.

What are some of the potential long-term implications of the development of sperm banks? Professor Rodney Harris explained:

> 'The most important long-term implication is the more effective management of infertility. Sperm may also be stored for men who are about to undergo treatment for cancer which is likely to damage the testes. Similarly, men who are likely to be carrying deleterious dominant genes may wish to store their sperm in the hope of future diagnostic tests or treatment. I am not impressed by fears that stored sperm might be used for "eugenic" purposes which has found little general favour.'

At present there is no effective control whatever in this country in the establishment of sperm banks and the commercialization of AID. There are however some indirect controls — professional NHS resources, for example.

Legal and Social Concerns of AIH: AID

The process of AID itself may be medically simple but it is fraught with legal and social complications which are more complex than at first apparent.

Legally children born by means of AID are defined as 'illegitimate', and the fact that the husband consents to AID is immaterial. Father usually enters his own name in the Birth Registration entry, in spite of the fact that this is actually to break the law and commit perjury (Registration Act 1965). In the past it might have been argued that the husband would not know that he was not the father should he have had intercourse during the month of insemination, or if his sperm was mixed with that of the donor's. The Royal College of Obstetricians and Gynaecologists[2] states that 'babies born within a marriage are presumed to be legitimate, and provided you do not abstain from intercourse during the period in which AID is carried out there can be no certainty that any child conceived is not your husband's'. Genetic tests are now able to prove whether the mother and her husband are likely to be the official biological parents. Some parents solve the problem by having another doctor deliver the child in ignorance of the facts of AID and they can therefore sign the certificate in good faith, but naturally the entry will be incorrect. The donor, and not the woman's husband, is the legal father.

At present the legal situation seems to be rather confused. A BMA working group (1983) recommended that the law should be changed to dispel any ambiguity of the legal status of the child born as a result of AID: thus, a child so born by means of AID to which the husband of the mother has consented in writing should be recognized as legitimate from the time of confirmation to conception.[3] The Law Society suggests consideration of a compulsory register of AID births, with discreet lettering as a code in the birth certificate.

The most important social implication of AID is that it affects the family structure. Some husbands find it difficult to come to terms with their own inadequacy to help produce a family, and feel that somehow they have failed in their manhood. The knowledge of their infertility comes to most men as a severe emotional and psychological shock, and is often mistakenly confused with impotency and lack of virility. Where AID is undertaken secretly and deliberately concealed from some family members, the basis of that trust, on which family relationships is essentially built, is undermined. Parents often find themselves caught up in a web of deceit, not only with their child but with the network of relatives. Yet such secrecy is sometimes seen as an advantage of AID over the alternative available to the infertile couple, namely adoption, and is advocated to combat the present legal situation so that the child is protected from the stigma of illegitimacy.

The majority, if not all, of the major reports[4] dealing with the practice of AID comment on the lack of evidence about its social consequences. In 1949 the Commission set up by the then Archbishop of Canterbury reported its findings. It recommended that AID should be considered to be a criminal offence, and in the House of Lords the Archbishop stated: 'My Committee observed, very truly, that as yet there is little evidence available upon which to judge the sociological and psychological affects of AID' (*Hansard* 1949, Vol. 161. No. 50, p. 40). The 1960 Feversham Committee which declared AID to be undesirable observed that, 'there is no doubt that all discussions of the practice is at present greatly handicapped by the lack of information about what has subsequently happened to the families of those women who have received AID'. Later, in 1973 the Peel Report, which was more favourably disposed to AID, affirmed: 'The Panel has had evidence from several sources urging that, for psychological reasons, there should be no follow-up of children born to AID. It understands but does not entirely agree with these views. Information must be obtained on the genetic effects, especially where frozen semen has been used it is important to learn the effects, in human terms, on the development of personal relationships in families resulting from the use of AID'.

The Report of the Royal College of Obstetricians and Gynaecologists (1976) also drew the attention to the lack of evidence of the social implications of AID. The Report (1979) of a working party set up under the auspices of the Free Church Federal Council and the British Council of Churches, confesses, 'We do not know what the long-term consequences of the social acceptance of AID will be.'

Such lack of evidence is mainly due to the atmosphere of secrecy which traditionally has surrounded the practice of AID. This was one of the factors mentioned by Professor Ian Kennedy:

> 'There are a number of failings in the normal studies of the whole subject of AID. It is an area which has been dogged by at least two problems. One is the secrecy of it all, which means that you cannot introduce all the relationships that are involved within the family. The other is the illegitimacy aspect of it, which stigmatizes it and makes it always look as though it's a second or third best way of having a family, and therefore causes parents to have a certain amount of guilt, and not produce an environment in which these open evaluations can be discussed. It is dogged by these and other factors that suggest that it is not really a nice thing to do'.

The social implications arise because AID affects the whole basis of family life. A family is artificially created by the use of semen donated by an anonymous third party, and for some AID families to keep such a long-term secret imposes a great deal of emotional stress and strain.

Should the AID child be able to know of his genetic origin? The majority of AID parents seem to keep the AID procedure secret from the child. In an explanatory information booklet for parents issued by the Royal College of Obstetricians and Gynaecologists (1979) it is stated: 'Unless you decide to tell the child there is no reason for him (or her) ever to know that he (or she) was conceived by AID. Whether or not you do so is entirely up to you'.[5] Advocates of disclosure say that the secret may be indirectly revealed in a family quarrel or break-up, but there seems no evidence that it does.

A Report of the Board of Social Responsibility (1983)

believes that telling children the truth may not necessarily involve revealing the identity of the donor. It would, however, require some information of a social and relational character. For this reason they recommend that (1) proper records should be kept, (2) deliberate policies designed to conceal the truth should not be followed, and (3) professional counselling support be made available to couples who choose this way forward to family life.[6]

Some assert that AID children have as much right to knowledge about their origins as have adopted children and see commitment to truth as a moral principle. There are advocates of the truth, too, who say that AID children ought to be told the truth not only because they may like to know but because they need to know. They should have a proper sense of who they are, for a person's identity is rooted in his or her biological make-up. To understand ourselves properly we need to know where we come from in the fullest sense of the word. Children might be told they were born through AID but need not be told the names of their biological fathers. Instead they would be allowed to have a kind of 'pen portrait' of the donor concerned with enough information to add up to a real 'image' in each instance. When I posed the question to the Dean of Durham, the Very Revd Peter Baelz, he stated:

> 'Yes. Questions of identity, "Who am I?", do include questions of biological parenthood. I think I should wish to know at least something about my biological father or mother. However, no one would give semen unless it was assumed that there would be complete confidentiality. I'm glad that the Board of Social Responsibility said that there ought to be some access to records, not to individual names. But that *is* a compromise, and perhaps an uneasy one.'

Professor Ian Kennedy considered it expedient first of all to separate out two reasons why a child might want to know:

> 'One reason might be to ascertain his true parentage and to know who the father was, and that, I think, poses problems, if only because it might mean that the donor of the sperm might be subjected later on to claims alleging

he has certain responsibilities to child support or whatever, because he would be identified as the parent. The effect of that might well be that donation of sperm would cease tomorrow. That would be one reason why you would be anxious to identify and it would be a reason which I think would be valid.

The other reason for knowing, which would not involve knowing the identity — in the sense of the name and address of the donor — would be so as to ascertain the genetic make up of oneself. If the person is asking us if there are some people whom he should not marry because, for example, the relationship would mean that the offspring would be genetically at risk, that is, the genetic offspring would have some impairment because the donor, for example, was the carrier of some factor which might put at risk any future children, this is, I think, information which the child ought to know. I have argued for the availability of a record which does not identify the donor but identifies the medical and scientific facts, which might be available to the child if and when the child might seek them. Now of course the child will only seek them if the child is aware of AID, and that is obviously a matter solely for the parents to resolve themselves.'

Others argue that AID children being told about their origin would have worse consequences than if they are being deceived. They support their viewpoint by the fact that among adopted children, who generally do know that the people who brought them up are not their real parents, very few go in search of their natural mothers and fathers. Under the 1975 Children Act, adopted people seeking access to their birth records must first undergo counselling by the Social Services. In 1982, 1684 people received such counselling. Almost all the subjects (1487) intended to apply for their birth certificates and 1191 desired further information from court records. Only 726, however, intended to try to trace their natural parents. The peak age for seeking information was the twenties and mid-thirties, probably because this is the time when adopted people would be raising families of their own.[7]

There are good medical reasons for the child to know that his mother's husband is not his genetic father. If his 'father' developed a familial disease the child might have unfounded anxiety that he also would develop it. Even worse, if it was a known heritable genetic disorder (e.g. Huntingdon's chorea, which does not reveal itself until later life) the child might decide against fathering any children himself for fear of passing on the disorder. Did Professor Ian Kennedy consider that any change in the law concerning the illegitimacy of an AID child was necessary?

'What is normally practised is some kind of illegality in that the husband of the mother is entered as the father which is technically incorrect and therefore a crime. It is more important to observe that illegitimacy as a state is, by and large, being eliminated by our law as having any significance. The difficulty is that it still has social significance and that the law cannot legislate social significance away. Therefore, merely to pass a law saying that the child should not be regarded as illegitimate may not solve the problem. I do however think that the law ought to change and I have tried to work out a way by which it could do so. I would concentrate on the form the official records would take.

I think that in the record of birth, the child should be entered as the child of the husband and mother, but with a special code accompanying this registration. This code should be known only to the registrars throughout the country and should contain the information that the child is an AID child. The registrar would then be able to recognize the code on any particular birth certificate and take account of, or reveal, as the case may be, the relevant AID information stored in a second register.'

The Donors
Generally in AID clinics sperm is obtained from medical students or volunteers who are either paid or unpaid for their services. They are normally chosen with care and screened for genetic abnormalities, although there are no laws which require these procedures. It is difficult to know how far to extend the choice of donors beyond general health, family history and physical characteristics. Most donors are largely

unknown quantities, hence some people's preference for using donors whose reproductive ability has been shown by the birth of normal children within marriage. Should a donor's wife be informed? Should the donor be paid a fee? Should he be accepted if proposed by the sterile couple? Who selects the donor? Sir Gordon Wolstenholme expressed his views on these questions as follows:

> 'I should prefer donations to be made only by single men. If a married man does donate, it would be intolerable if this were not done in consultation with his wife. When blood donors are paid they tend to conceal a past history of illness which would exclude them. The semen donor is put to some trouble, with blood and sample tests, history and interview, and some modest compensation does not seem to be unreasonable.
> No. I think he should always be anonymous.
> An experienced fertility clinic.'

What did the Dean of Durham see as some of the problems posed by the donor, the 'third party'?

> 'I am concerned that a person donates semen but refuses all responsibility for the consequent child.
>
> You could say that a donor is doing a service to childless couples by making it possible for them to have a child. This could be a form of altruism, and on purely consequentialist grounds you might argue that it is a good thing. However, on non-consequentialist grounds you might raise questions of responsibility. Is it perhaps inhuman to give semen but not to be concerned about what happens afterwards?
>
> We have to ask what responsibilities are we called to accept in the whole process of procreation. It is not simply a giving of semen; it is not just caring for a mother who is pregnant; it is not just producing a child. It is also bringing that child up and giving it a name and an identity.'

Donor selection needs reappraisal and motivations deserve serious consideration.[8] Czyba and Manuel (1981) outline a disciplined practice of AID in France where in a number of hospital centres only frozen semen is used. No payment is

made for semen donation, making it a free gift. Semen is taken
only from married donors who are also fathers, with the full
consent of their wives.

It is important that records be kept of the donors, not least
because of the need to avoid incest. There is always the
possibility of a donor's 'children' (half-brothers and half-
sisters) meeting and unwittingly marrying. Also some couples
might wish to have a number of children from the same donor.
The evidence of the Law Society reveals that where doctors or
others offer artificial insemination on a large scale with semen
of concealed or unidentified origin, the prospects of half-
brothers and sisters meeting and mating increase almost
exponentially. A recent study undertaken by Curie-Cohen
(1979) shows most physicians never use a donor for more than
six pregnancies, but in one instance a single donor was used
for fifty pregnancies.[9] If the same donor is responsible for a
limited number of conceptions the actual risk of incest is very
small, for if 2,000 live children a year were to be born in
Britain as a result of AID, and each donor were to be
responsible for five children, an unwitting incestuous marriage is unlikely to take place more than once in fifty to one
hundred years.[10]

Interchange of semen between centres is one solution. Ice-
land (population circa 300,000) has a very active AID
programme using donor semen from Scandanavia and Denmark.

The practice of providing AID for single women and lesbian couples is already a reality, albeit in isolated instances.
The growing recognition of 'women's right to choose' indicates that the demand is likely to increase, particularly since
adoption can be made on the application of one person alone
(Children Act 1975: 5.11). Also as there are now available
'home insemination kits', complete with sperm and instructions for use, it seems difficult to regulate the practice.[11] Such
procedures raise serious implications for the child and also the
family as the basic unit of society. They also create major legal
and ethical problems.

Ethical Concerns of AIH:AID.

AIH as a therapy seems to raise few if any ethical problems, and appears justifiable on christian grounds where it is used to bring about conception which cannot otherwise be achieved. From a moral standpoint AIH, is a totally different issue from AID, and it is over the latter rather than the former that the ethical debate is conducted. To some people masturbation may seem aesthetically distasteful or morally reprehensible, although in these incidences it ought not to be confused with the seeking of solitary erotic pleasure, but directed solely towards procreation. In the moral teaching of the Roman Catholic Church AIH:AID is officially rejected.[12]

Non-Roman Catholic churches take a far more tolerant view toward AIH, accepting masturbation when it is the only way an otherwise sterile couple can achieve procreation.[13] There are also a number of Roman Catholic theologians who share this viewpoint (Haring *et al*).

Although some agree that AID can bring fulfilment and happiness to an otherwise infertile marriage, there are others who maintain that donor semen represents an 'adulteration' of the whole marriage relationship. Yet it is extremely difficult to sustain an argument that AID is an act of adultery for there is no physical contact, and consent has been given by both parties. To hold acts of AID adulterous as to doctor, wife, or donor, may lead to absurd results since the doctor may be a woman, or the husband himself may administer the insemination; to consider it an act of adultery with the donor who at the time of insemination may be thousands of miles away, or may even be dead, is equally absurd.[14]

It is the act of intervention by an anonymous and non-responsible third person, or 'intruder', into procreation in marriage which causes some concern in AID, for the biological bond between husband and wife is severed and the marriage covenant violated. There would, however, be those who would not acknowledge any violation of the marriage bond if both husband and wife have consented to the procedure.

The Lambeth Conference (1958) agreed that artificial insemination by anyone other than the husband raised problems of such gravity that the committee could not see any possibility of its acceptance by Christian people. Such views were reaffirmed by the 1968 Lambeth Conference.

The Report, *Choices in Childlessness*, (1982) expressed the view (of some of its members) that there is a specifically christian objection to the practice of AID. Their objection rests 'on the conviction that marriage is a covenant-relationship between husband and wife exclusive of all others, not only in sexual intercourse, but also in the procreation of children. If there is going to be a child by the one, then so long as the covenant relationship endures, it shall be a child by both; if it is not to be by both, then it shall be by neither. This is part of the meaning of a marriage "for better for worse"' (p. 43).

The technique of artificial insemination also introduces a number of alternatives which give rise to further ethical and legal dilemmas (see p.185). Freezing and storage of sperm may be used to impregnate a woman, other than the wife, but with the wife's consent, who then acts as a 'host' mother. Sperm may also be stored by the husband prior to vasectomy, including its usage after his death. An additional indication for long term storage is when the husband has a malignancy requiring drugs or radiotherapy (e.g. seminoma of the testes). Again a woman can be inseminated by sperm which is other than her husband's.

It is not to be denied that AID, which is practised widely, brings much joy and fulfilment to many a marriage, but it does need to be subject to much stricter social, ethical and legal safeguards than it appears to have at present.

In Vitro Fertilization
The fertilization of a human egg in a laboratory and its implantation and growth in the mother's womb was first successfully achieved in Britain on 25 July 1978, with the birth of the world's first test-tube baby, Louise Brown, delivered by Mr Patrick Steptoe at Oldham General Hospital. This technique by which a woman's egg is fertilized by her husband's sperm is known scientifically as '*in vitro* fertilization' (*in vitro* meaning 'in glass'). Some hundreds of babies have now been born '*in vitro*' throughout the world (Australia, France, USA, Sweden and Denmark), and the technique is being used in many more centres worldwide. In Britain Mr Steptoe and Dr Robert Edwards now run a private clinic at Bourn Hall, Cambridge, where more than 439 'clinical' pregnancies have

been established and 215 babies born (May 1984).

Other IVF programmes are held at Cromwell Hospital, London, Hammersmith Hospital, St Mary's Hospital, Manchester, and elsewhere. The success rate in obtaining a continuing pregnancy by this particular method of production is reported to be between ten and twenty per cent, and this figure is expected to rise to about thirty per cent in the near future. By 1981 *in vitro* fertilization had been established as a clinical procedure.[15]

Infertile couples undergo a very high level of anxiety. A recent study at the Royal Free Hospital (Johnston 1984) revealed that women were as anxious as they would be if facing major surgery. Pressures also come from the natural instinct for procreation, responsibility to the partner, pressures from members of the family and acquaintances.

In vitro fertilization (IVF) was developed by Mr Patrick Steptoe, a gynaecologist of Oldham, and Dr Robert Edwards, a biologist of Cambridge, to overcome infertility, or inability to conceive, in women whose fallopian tubes are irremediably blocked, have been damaged beyond repair by previous disease, or in whom surgical intervention of one kind or another has left them with inadequate tubal function (estimated some 20,000 in Britain). The ova are removed from the woman's ovaries around the time of ovulation. Egg production can often be more readily controlled, and subsequently egg collection rendered more reliable, by giving the woman hormone injections to stimulate egg production. Surgeons find the follicles in which there are ripe eggs by inserting a laparoscope — a telescope which carries its own light — through a small abdominal incision. The follicles are punctured with a special needle and the eggs and their fluid are sucked out directly into the test-tubes. They are then fertilized with the husband's semen in a culture medium, and placed in a special incubator kept at blood heat. The sperm swim around the egg until one finally penetrates the egg's outer shell. This is the process of conception which, by some definitions, constitutes the beginning of human life.

Each fertilized egg has two half sets of chromosomes, one from the father and one from the mother, which fuse to form a single nucleus. After fertilization the egg begins to divide rapidly into two, four, then eight cells, with the chromosomes in each cell carrying the genes for potentially normal development to a normal baby. The embryo is usually implanted in the uterus when it reaches the eight-cell stage — some two or three days after fertilization. The embryo implant is a minor surgical procedure. Cell division then proceeds. The embryo becomes attached to the wall of the uterus, and after eight to nine weeks the separate organs of the body will have developed to reach the fetal stage.

There is an alternative method which is being used which does not involve fertilization outside the mother's body. The egg and semen are transferred back immediately so that fertilization then takes place in the uterus. Advocates of this method claim that if their simplified method can be modified to yield results as good as the present method then the management of infertility will come within the compass of local hospitals.

An improved technique has recently been developed (King's College Hospital) in which the procedure can be done in an out-patient department. The ovaries of the patient are first stimulated by the giving of a hormone (FSH). A second hormone (HCG) precipitates ovulation, and thirty-five hours afterwards a woman is ready to have three or four ova aspirated from her ovary. Fifty hours later the patient returns to have the fertilized eggs, embryos, implanted in her uterus. No anaesthetics are needed and costs are considerably reduced. As yet the procedure has produced no side effects, but it has to be carried out by members of a highly trained team.

Obstetricians now have much more control over 'test-tube' pregnancies than normal ones. Women can choose whether to have one, or two, or three eggs implanted in the uterus. Multiple implantations increase the chances of pregnancy, and implanting more than one egg does not necessarily lead to the birth of twins. Two eggs would give the mother a better chance of producing a successful pregnancy. The implanting of one embryo gives sixteen per cent of pregnancies, two gives twenty-five per cent, and three results in thirty per cent. It is common for twins to be born and this often offers an extra bonus to an older mother. However, the increased physical risks to the mother, and the outcome of pregnancy with multiple pregnancies have to be emphasized. These risks of multiple pregnancy must be balanced against the risks involved in waiting to repeat the process, possibly including laparoscopy, during a subsequent cycle. Fifty to seventy per cent of embryos once implanted go on to develop into babies, and a woman treated by 'test-tube' techniques has a fifteen to twenty per cent chance of giving birth to a healthy baby. There is great joy when IVF is successful, but the failures are sometimes forgotten. The stress of repeated attempts, as well as the financial cost, can impose considerable strain on the couple. Improvements are mostly needed in the replanting of the embryos, for this remains the major stumbling block to higher rates of successful pregnancies.

Surrogate Mothers and Womb Leasing

The term 'surrogate mother', that is, a person who, for financial or compassionate reasons, agrees to bear a child for someone else, is applied to two different situations. In the one instance the 'surrogate' or 'substitute' herself contributes the ova which are fertilized with the sperm of the male partner, naturally or by artificial insemination. This procedure is also described as 'egg donation', which would be akin to AID. The second example is where the surrogate provides the womb into which is implanted the embryo of the childless couple, which has been fertilized *in vitro*. The child would then be returned to its genetic parents after delivery. This type of surrogate motherhood is commonly known as 'womb leasing', if the mother is to be paid to carry the pregnancy. This would make it possible for a couple to 'have' a child which would be totally biologically their own without the child's 'mother' ever giving birth. Surrogate motherhood might well be used when a woman suffers from a severe heart disease, partial paralysis, has a history of frequent miscarriages, or is the carrier of an hereditary disease. Another possible use for surrogate motherhood is the instance where the mother does not wish to carry the child because it interferes with her career, and so serves as a mere convenience.

Freezing of Human Embryos (Cryostorage)

In Melbourne, Australia, and in the UK doctors are now

freezing embryos which can be thawed out when needed and implanted in the patient's womb at just the right point in her monthly cycle. This would of course greatly simplify the donation of embryos. In addition, if freezing were to be used along with fertility drugs, it could also reduce the present high failure rate for couples using their own ova and sperm. It would mean that women who had failed to have a 'test-tube' baby at the first attempt could try again without undergoing a second egg collection operation. It would also enable women to have an IVF pregnancy months or even years after they or their partners had been sterilized, or even after their husband's death. There is the possibility that prior to freezing and implantation the embryo might be checked for any genetic disorders. R. G. Edwards (1981) observes that 'identifying embryos with genetic abnormalities would offer an alternative to amniocentesis during the second trimester of pregnancy, and the "abortion *in vitro*" of a defective preimplantation embryo, still free-living, minute and undifferentiated, would be infinitely preferable to abortion *in vivo* at twenty weeks of pregnancy or thereabouts as the results of amniocentesis are obtained. It would also be less traumatic for parents and doctor to type several embryos and replace or store those that are normal rather than having the threat of a mid-term abortion looming over each successive pregnancy.'[16]

The world's first baby from a frozen embryo was born by caesarian section on 28 March 1984, at Melbourne's Queen Victoria Medical Centre. Zoe, a 5lb 13oz girl, was born after the embryo had been frozen for eight weeks at −196°C. Her birth marks a major advance in the laboratory control of human reproduction, and raises major legal and ethical problems for society. Zoe's mother was treated in the Medical Centre's *in vitro* fertilization programme, in which ten of her eggs were fertilized and three resulting embryos were transplanted into her uterus. She did not become pregnant and six of the seven remaining embryos developed normally and were frozen in liquid nitrogen three days after fertilization. Two months later, in another attempt at pregnancy, three embryos were thawed and transferred to her uterus. One attached itself to the uterus lining. Although premature, the child was healthy and began breastfeeding almost immediately. The freeze-thaw process has important implications for *in vitro* fertilized births, reducing the risk of multiple pregnancies and the number of operations required to retrieve eggs.

The Melbourne team has at present some two hundred embryos frozen in storage. Soon many thousands will be stored all over the world. Guidelines drawn up by the Australian National Health and Medical Research Council Ethics Committee stipulate that such frozen embryos should not be stored for more than ten years, although it might be possible to store them indefinitely.

Future Research

The present developments in the sphere of *in vitro* fertilization in the United Kingdom give little rise for concern. What is disturbing is the possibility of future developments, for on the near horizon are the possibilities of the use of donor oocytes and embryos for infertile women, the use of surrogate mothers and the deliberate selection of embryos of one sex in the case of specific sex-linked diseases such as haemophilia and muscular dystrophy.

1. Experimentation with embryos: There are a number of scientists who wish to carry out research on 'spare' embryos or indeed to fertilize human eggs simply for research purposes. Test-tube baby pioneers face the dilemma whether they should destroy a specimen or preserve the minute bundle of cells and observe the process of embryonic growth for as long as possible. In his recent publication, *Human Conception In Vitro*,[17] Dr Edwards points out that identifying genetic defects in embryos would offer a preferable alternative to testing mothers in mid-pregnancy and having to perform abortions. It is stated that embryonic research would also provide invaluable insights into how the organs of the body develop and why they sometimes develop abnormally. Such research would help doctors understand and therefore eventually prevent genetic defects. Dr Edwards himself admits that the prospect poses a considerable ethical dilemma.

At present the Medical Research Council has given permission for embryos to be preserved up to the age of fourteen days.

2. *'Cloning'* is a botanical term meaning cutting. A plant grown from a cutting is cloned; it grows into a new plant having identical characteristics with its parent. In this process the nucleus of an ovum is removed and replaced by the nucleus of an asexual cell (i.e. a skin cell) with the production of a being genetically identical to the donor of the nucleus. Human beings who are replicas of one another and carbon copies of individuals would be produced. Cloning has already proved possible with varying success in sheep, frogs, salamanders, and fruit flies; it has not yet been successful in higher animals or man. The male partner would be no longer necessary for this asexual form of reproduction, for all members of a clone are of the same sex. Mothers and fathers would be able to generate sons and daughters genetically identical to themselves.

3. *Choosing the sex of offspring:* IVF, cloning and freezing techniques could be used to establish the sex of the embryo before it is returned to the mother's uterus. Women would be able to be offered female pregnancies should they carry the genes for haemophilia or muscular dystrophy, diseases in which only boys are affected, and for which at present women who do carry these genes are offered the opportunity of therapeutic abortion of their male babies. At the present time ultrasound or amniocentesis followed by chromosomal analysis is able to identify the sex of the foetus as early as sixteen to eighteen weeks gestation. These procedures however can only be used at a relatively late stage of pregnancy. Should a fetus of the affected gender be identified Section 1.1B of the Abortion Act allows a late abortion to be carried out. Only one in two males would be affected, for fifty per cent of male abortions are normal fetuses.

The new technique of chorion biopsy, which is a method of obtaining a fragment of placental tissue using suction on a fine catheter passed through the cervix, enables a definite diagnosis of some disorders (e.g. muscular dystrophy) to be made (as well as fetal sex) by eight to ten weeks. This is a rapidly progressing field but not yet universally available. The risk of abortion following this procedure is at present much greater than after amniocentesis.

4. Ectogenesis: Ectogenesis refers to the entire growth of the embryo and fetus outside the human body. This of course does occur for a short period of time at present during the procedure of IVF when after fertilization the very early embryo of two cells is grown in a medium in the laboratory. Very small premature babies of less than 1000g are at present being kept alive in incubators in some neonatal intensive care nurseries.

Babies may be born prematurely, (or abort late), because there is something wrong with them or with the uterus. In other instances (e.g. severe hypertension) they are delivered electively because the chances of survival in the womb are slender and there are significant maternal risks. The increasing skills of the paediatricians in keeping these little 'abortuses' alive means that for many babies a point is reached where the SCBU (Special Care Baby Unit) is a safer container for them than the uterus. No artificial placenta has yet been successfully designed to support fetal life in the first half of pregnancy. Ectogenesis would save the lives of many babies who at present die of extreme prematurity after miscarriage or premature labour.

5. Genetic manipulation: An important aspect of 'genetic engineering' is the scope for 'gene therapy' in the treatment of an individual with genetic disease. Such therapy entails the permanent genetic modification of human cells with DNA containing the required gene or genes. Gene manipulation could produce permanent physical or psychological damage to the child if techniques were faulty. Also such manipulations might well result in a normal child but with an altered constitution.

A recent WHO (World Health Organization) Report stated that there are over one hundred million carriers for potentially lethal inherited blood diseases such as stickle cell anaemia and thalassaemia, and approximately 200,000 affected children die each year from this simple set of gene defects. At present it is not possible to carry out gene therapy, but, nevertheless, the way in which it might be developed either on early embryos or on individual patients is clear in outline from research now in progress.

6. *Human-animal hybrids:* It may be possible in future to create man-animal hybrids by inserting human genetic material into an egg cell of an animal. The usage of egg cells of primates would be more likely to achieve success because of their closer evolutionary relationship to humans. Such creatures it has been suggested might be employed in undertaking demeaning and dangerous jobs, and so protect human beings from danger and hazardous unpleasant occupations.[18]

Legal and Social Concerns of IVF

Dr Robert Edwards in his Horizon Lecture (1983) stated that those involved in the work of *in vitro* fertilization often have to make complex decisions against an obscure and often confused legal, social and ethical background. At present there seems almost no effective legal control of IVF and no specific laws dealing with test-tube children. Indeed such legislation may be viewed as an undesirable intrusion into the sphere of clinical practice.[19]

The Royal College of Obstetricians and Gynaecologists recommend that legislation be enacted to register directors of institutions where IVF and ER (embryo replacement) is being carried out and also to license the premises. Secretaries of State should have power on the advice of a statutory body to make regulations: (1) to license and inspect premises where IVF and ER are carried out: (2) to register directors of institutions where these procedures are performed: (3) to forbid both (a) IVF and ER (b) experiments on human embryos, to be carried out other than under the direction of registered persons in licensed premises.[20] It is desirous, too, for careful follow-up studies to be carried out on all babies conceived *in vitro*.

The nature of the family, of inheritance, and even of individual identity itself, are not least among the legal and social questions raised in 'test-tube baby' work. What are some of the main areas of concern?

1. One important sphere of potential social concern is that IVF provides an additional means of separating '*love-making*' from '*life*'- or '*baby-making*', and procreation from sexual intercourse.[21] Some critics would argue that there is a danger of turning human reproduction into a laboratory process. For example, Paul Ramsey (1970) bases his argument on two scriptural passages both of which emphasize the basis of love and the sanctity of marriage (St John 1. 1–15: Ephesians 5), and affirms that to put asunder what God has joined together in parenthood when he made love procreative, to procreate beyond the sphere of love (AID, for example, or making human life in a test-tube), or to posit acts of sexual love beyond the sphere of responsible creation (by definition, marriage), means a refusal of the image of God's creation in our own.[22] Pope Pius XII condemned artificial insemination as immoral and absolutely unlawful, because it separated the love-giving and life-giving elements of married life, and in a letter to *The Times*, (12 February 1982), the then Bishop of Durham (the present Archbishop of York) emphasized the close link between the physical and the personal as the very feature of our humanity. Robert Morrison, in *The Biological Time Bomb*, states that 'once sex and reproduction are separated, society will have to struggle with defining the nature of interpersonal relationships which have no long-term social point . . . and seek new ways to ensure reasonable care for infants and children in an emotional atmosphere which lacks biological reinforcement.'[23]

On the other hand there are those who advocate that the act of sexual intercourse is no guarantee to a happy and healthy family environment, and that the process of *in vitro* fertilization demands sacrifice on the part of both husband and wife far beyond anything required for normal procreation. At Bourn Hall, Cambridge, Dr Robert Edwards emphasized this very point:

> 'I have long suspected arguments that conception *in vivo* expresses "love", whereas fertilization *in vitro* debases it. The loving demands of infertile couples, one to the other,

during fertilization *in vitro* can be far greater than during a chance sexual act leading to conception.'

He refers (1974) to the fact that bodily love is already removed from procreation by means of a number of contraceptive devices, and questions how the withholding of treatment from the infertile can be countenanced against the notion of family life which has survived abortion, divorce, sexual freedom, and rejection of the parents by their children.[24] Professor Oliver O'Donovan found himself a little ambivalent on the particular issue of the technological separation of conception from sexual intercourse:

'My answer is not dogmatic and decisive about this. I want to say first of all that there is a clear *prima facie* commitment in Christian understanding of marriage to keep together the procreative and unitive functions of marriage and of sexual intercourse, and not to take one apart from the other in such a way that childbearing becomes a *project* that you are engaged in, a technical project which has nothing whatsoever to do with your married life. Clearly it seems to me that psychologically and emotionally the relation to the child interacts with the relationship of the couple to each other, and this is one of the beauties of human conception.

   Nevertheless, having said that the unitive and procreative ends go together in Christian understanding of marriage, there's a flexibility about that "going together". As Anglicans we have never accepted the conservative Roman Catholic act-analysis of that going together which says that in every single sexual act there has to be openness to procreation. . . . Clearly, what you are doing if you take the actual moment of conception away from the natural intercourse and do it *in vitro*, is putting another strain on this principle of holding the procreative and the unitive together.'

He still thought there was a problem about separating the conception from the union of the husband and wife.

'But it seems to me that if this is the only way which a couple can become parents in this sense, then it's acceptable, though not obviously the best way. I don't think it's an absolutely clear case of something that shouldn't be done; on the other hand I do think it's a clear case of something that has enormous social dangers.'

The question that the Church should be considering, and one very much in the mind of the Very Revd Peter Baelz is, 'What do we believe to be the desirable norm for having children?' and he offered some personal thoughts.

> 'I myself would want it to be a continuing responsibility in which the physical, the emotional, and the spiritual are united, so that the norm will be the physical begetting of children and the sharing in bringing them up. Now, when you move away from that norm because some things are not working, at each move you have to justify an exception in which there is greater good than harm. However, if you simply analyse the whole process into a number of separate acts so that someone gives a sperm and someone else gives an ovum, and another person provides a womb, and so you put together a child, then, however much the child will be loved, you are breaking up the unity and wholeness of the process of procreation. Procreation needs a kind of wholeness which, if we divide it into a number of separate parts, we are in danger of losing. What is it that makes a human life human? This is the question. Surely it is something which is reflected in the continuing care and responsibility which produced life and nurtures it into a full humanity.'

As the infertile couple are of themselves incapable of producing a child by the normal means of sexual intercourse and are prepared to make sacrifices to overcome a physical defect, IVF may be seen as an appropriate use of technology, ('inferior' as it is to one involving the bodies and personalities of two individuals), rather than as a dehumanizing factor to their family life. It seems fitting to enable a stable married couple to remedy their childlessness by means of an egg from the mother (and not another woman), and sperm preferably from the husband (if this is impossible then sperm from an anonymous donor). It is to be hoped that it will only be resorted to as a therapy to rectify such a defect, and that couples be advised to undergo counselling, not only throughout the period of investigation and treatment, but also afterwards.

2. *The deep-freezing of embryos:* This raises obvious fundamental social, legal and ethical issues. A successful pregnancy would show that any embryo taken from one generation could, technically, be reanimated in the next. Again, no one knows if the very process of freezing may cause damage to an embryo in the short or long-term. Neither is it possible to be certain that those individuals born as a result of deeply frozen embryos may not become victims of a latent defect. This was the guiding moral line taken by Professor Ian Kennedy:

> 'With freezing there are several problems. First, freezing for the purpose of whom? If it is done in order to give the woman, whose ovum it was, another chance of pregnancy on a subsequent occasion, rather than have to go over the process again, then there is no question of the problem of surrogate motherhood arising. I regard this as utterly repugnant because I do not think it is in the interest of any child to be exposed to possible competition as to motherhood between a uterine mother and a natural mother. But when you freeze for the purpose of the mother, then there shouldn't be any difficulties. There should not be any objections for it is the same as IVF. But there is one major difficulty, namely that you have to demonstrate that the freezing process does not cause the fetus any harm. Any analysis of IVF must adhere to the principle that you may not do anything that is not in the best interests of the child. That is the guiding moral line. You cannot freeze it, and later implant it, if risks exist that it will be genetically harmed.'

The question then arises, How are we to demonstrate that there will be no risks of genetic disablement by this freezing process?

> 'The answer can only be by doing it! But the difficulty is that by doing it, you may in fact expose a child to genetic

disablement. Therefore, one may take the absolutist view that you may not therefore do it. I happen to find this view persuasive. The intention of the researcher has also to be examined. If you freeze with the purpose later on of doing research, then I think you fall foul, on my analysis, of the arguments I have been putting forward previously about the intention of a researcher being to use that which could have been implanted as a means to an end rather than an end itself, worthy of respect.'

Professor Ian Craft did not see the freezing of embryos as an illogical concept if it is considered to be an aspect of assisting an individual couple achieve their ability to become pregnant:

'Situations may arise whereby a woman receives drugs to induce ovulation and a number of eggs result. If, for example, one obtained six eggs and all of these fertilized, it may not be sensible to transfer all six embryos just in case the patient may have a triplet or quadruplet pregnancy which produces obstetric problems. Therefore one could consider giving the patient two chances to become pregnant if three embryos were used on one occasion, and three stored for a short period of time to be inserted into the uterus after the first pregnancy was completed, if a pregnancy resulted, or after a few months if the first embryo transfer did not succeed.

I personally think it would be sensible to put a time limit on the duration of storage, and three to five years might be a sensible time. There obviously may be anxiety that the freezing process may have an adverse effect on development, but there is no evidence in work undertaken in animals to indicate there is any increased abnormality of liveborn young following successful *in vitro* fertilization using frozen embryos.'

The problem of freezing embryos for later use has split the medical profession itself.

The Royal College of General Practitioners (1983) lists the freezing of human embryos as unethical. The Royal College of Obstetricians and Gynaecologists (1983) on the other hand approve the procedure. They are of the opinion that, in the light of the considerable animal experience already available, it would be justified in endorsing cryostorage of embryos in the hope of improving the success rate of IVF and ER. They recommend an initial limitation of the storage time to that required for a foreseeable and specific purpose, e.g. a second pregnancy to the same couple. Such an arbitrary time limit is suggested on social rather than on scientific grounds and to avoid unpredictable legal hazards.[25] The Royal Society also generally welcomes the use of cryostorage, while the working party of the BMA recommends that cryostorage should not exceed twelve months and should be done on behalf of a particular patient/couple.

There is no known limit to the time human embryos can be preserved: animal studies show that mouse embryos can be thawed after five years and develop normally. Its application to humans, however, is not the same as its application to mice or cattle. As Grobstein (1982) comments: 'Ninety per cent success rates may be acceptable for laboratory and domestic animals. In humans it is the ten per cent failure rate that is of concern — particularly if these are partial failures, not detectable until after birth or even later in life. Clearly these are matters for most careful consideration before frozen-thawed human embryos are reinserted for continued development.'[26]

Trounson and Mohr (1983) state that if the survival periods of frozen embryos approach the number of years observed in other animals difficulties may arise if parents disagree on their eventual destination. They suggest that patients may be asked to include in their wills their preferences concerning the destination of embryos in case of death. Options may include the donation of embryos to couples where both husband and wife are sterile, or it may be considered that the patients have the right to dispose of the embryos.[27]

At present there is no proper enforcement of legislation over the use of cryostorage, and many social and legal issues arise. Who is to have access to them? What would happen to them if their parents were to die or be divorced? Are possibly hundreds of human embryos to be kept in a freezer storage for long periods? What is the status of the embryo? A long-term storage of frozen embryos and their later thawing for implantation might easily create a number of emotional family

traumas, as well as legal questions of legitimacy and maintenance orders.

3. Surrogate motherhood and womb-leasing: There are already a
few babies in Britain who have been brought into the world by
means of surrogate mothers. The Law Society defines womb
leasing as 'the deliberate engineering of an illegitimate child
with the intention (whether disavowed or not) that it be
available for future adoption by a couple including either the
genetic father or the genetic mother of the child. Any contact
for the natural insemination by a man of a woman leasing her
womb for the purpose of bearing his child is almost certainly
illegal (in the sense that is will be unenforceable) because a
contract for sexual intercourse is against public policy'. It
recommends that if it is illegal, and probably criminal, for
people to deal commercially in children, it is worth
considering whether the time has come when it should become criminal for: (a) a woman to offer, for reward of any
kind, to bear a child for another person: (b) a man or a woman
to offer such a reward to a woman: (c) a person to act as an
agent or intermediary in such a transaction.

There are formidable dangers of emotional trauma when
the surrogate mother does not wish to give up the baby at
birth to the genetic mother. She may change her mind and
decide, for example, to abort the pregnancy or to keep the
child herself. An initial agreement to give up the child is not
an enforceable legal contract. The legal mother is the 'person
from whose body the baby emerges.' The surrogate mother
cannot be compelled to hand the baby back to the intended
parents. In any case there will probably be deep distress at
having to part with the baby she has carried for nine months.
If the baby is born with a deformity both genetic and surrogate mothers might wish to reject the child and this could lead
to a variety of legal problems. All these risks can be com-
pounded by the effect of commercialization.

There have been instances where couples have been
advertising to find surrogates for money, and such a practice
has prompted some people to set up in business selling the
services of surrogates. Such economic exploitation creates
moral, social and legal confusion, as well as psychological

harm to the surrogate mothers, the prospective adoptive parents, and the children concerned. It also introduces the idea of a 'contract' in which the baby is reduced from a human being and becomes something resembling a product. Little wonder, therefore, that surrogate motherhood has been described as 'a potential legal minefield'. Although it is often considered as the equivalent of AID, it is not. There are significant physical and psychological hazards for the surrogate mother which do not exist for the semen donor.

There is little doubt that womb leasing could become a solution for some childless couples. It might be argued that a woman or close relative might quite voluntarily offer her help to a couple who otherwise would be childless. Such a proposition would be an intimate personal offering made on behalf of another with the best of motives.

A recent case (April 1983) was reported where an identical twin, with identical genetic codes to her sister, bore a child on her behalf, after being inseminated with her sister's husband's semen. This however might well be only one factor in the situation. The months of bearing and nourishing the child create a bonding relationship and the handing over of the child when born might prove intolerable. It would be somewhat analagous to the factors which make it undesirable for an unmarried mother to arrange for the *immediate* adoption of her child. In the instance quoted above both sisters were soon to discover just what an emotional maelstrom they had created for themselves.

Although such an act of sisterly love might not involve the degradation of 'commercialization', one approaches instead the problems of incest and near-incest. The procedure is fraught with emotional complications and represents an unwise interference with the most sensitive fabric of the mother-child relationship. Medically of course it is an uncomplicated and low-risk procedure, but it carries with it serious moral and legal implications. It would seem to reduce procreation to nothing more than a biological process. Professor Ian Craft expressed his reservations:

'I find this a very difficult area to entertain for obvious reasons. There are indeed few medical reasons why it should be considered. One possibility could be the situation whereby a woman is born without a uterus, but has a normal genetal tract and whose ovaries regularly ovulate each month. Whilst this situation deserves considerable sympathy, the consequences of surrogate motherhood can be so profound that I feel that the Government enquiry is likely to suggest that this is not practised.'

The British Medical Association has recommended that doctors should have no involvement with any scheme advocating surrogate mothers. The central ethical committee of the BMA (March 1984) recommends that doctors should not become involved in any procedure in which a woman bears a child for another woman and then hands it over after birth, whether the treatment is done privately or even if it were to be attempted on the National Health Service with no fees involved. The committee is also opposed to such treatment whether it is undertaken by artificial insemination or by the test-tube baby technique. Once a woman was pregnant, however, doctors would have an obvious duty to care for her and the baby.

4. Predetermination of sex: The parental selection of the sex of their child might well raise major social problems. The sex ratio might become grossly imbalanced, one way or the other, resulting in acute social consequences. Embryos of the sex not desired might also be discarded or donated to another prospective parents.

Ethical Concerns of IVF
Are new ethical rules now needed to scrutinize the recently acquired ability of scientists to manipulate the beginnings of human life? In his *Brave New World Revisited* (1958), Aldous Huxley wrote: 'The prophecies made in 1931 (*Brave New World*) are coming true much sooner than I thought they would'. At present there is a diverse body of opinion both in the theological, scientific, and medical worlds, for the legal, ethical and scientific possibilities resulting from IVF and associated research prompt a great deal of debate and controversy. The various reports submitted to the Warnock Com-

mittee show that while some groups are totally opposed to the whole concept of IVF, others welcome it as a treatment for infertility while reserving judgement on such issues as the freezing of embryos and womb leasing. While there seem few if any objections to test-tube fertilization as long as it involves only the childless couple, the situation is very different regarding the other four methods of artificial reproduction, AID, egg donation, womb leasing and surrogate motherhood. These all depend on the involvement of a third party and this raises serious objections in the minds of many people.

Professor Ian Craft expressed his views on sperm and/or ovum donation in reply to the questions, What is the role of sperm, or indeed ovum, donation with this particular technique? Should there be a place to consider both sperm and ovum donation for an individual couple?

> 'There will be some couples who seek *in vitro* fertilization in whom the husband has no sperm, and I personally feel it is justified to use donor sperm in these circumstances as we currently do in patients who have various forms of infertility where part of the problem is the failure of the husband to produce sperm. Similarly there is a small group of women in whom there is a distinct risk that, if they become pregnant, the child might have a chance of an inheritance disorder, and in these circumstances one would appreciate their desire to have an egg donated to them by another person on a voluntary basis.'

He saw no difference in principle between ovum and sperm donation.

> 'However, I would recommend that there would be advantages if these developments in modern medical practice might be undertaken within a hospital environment where there is an ethical committee to ensure confidentiality of records, patient consent etc.
>
> The same would apply if ever a situation were to arise where both sperm and ovum donation might be considered in a particular couple both of whom had particular problems. Although no one is entertaining this idea at the moment, one can appreciate those adopting

children after birth who, on questioning, state that they would have preferred to adopt an embryo where possible just to experience the pleasure of pregnancy and child-birth. If this practice was ever sanctioned, it would raise important issues which are currently being considered by the Department of Health and Social Security enquiry. I personally feel that the woman who would give birth to such a child would indeed be the mother, irrespective of the source of the original genetic material.'

Again, there are those who would not see infertility as a disease in the sense that it interferes in an organic sense with the everyday life of the individual concerned, and consider that the psychological state associated with the inability to produce children might be overcome by an acceptance of the condition of infertility. They ask, is it justifiable therefore to use such procedures to satisfy the desire to have children? Is it a fitting use of the human reproductive power, of our sexu-ality? Is childlessness an insuperable handicap or disability?

I put the question to Professor Ian Craft: Does IVF fall within the normal prerogatives of the practice of medicine in the sense that it is satisfying the desires of human beings rather than practising the art or science of healing? He saw it as practising the art of healing

'inasmuch as those affected by infertility are frequently very emotionally upset by their problem, and it also satisfies the demands of patients whether the result of treatment is successful or not, in that they feel that everything is being done to achieve their objective. I think society has unfortunately given too little attention to the childless, and many of those who appear particularly critical of recent developments of treating infertility, particularly by *in vitro* fertilization, usually have a happy family of their own and are unaffected by the problem.'

There are of course good reasons to oppose any uncritical claims to the 'right' to reproduce children. The principal consideration should always be given to the child's welfare rather than the adult's desire, for we are dealing with a desire which leads to the creation of a new individual who also has rights. Doubts sometimes arise as to whether all women who want to avail themselves of these procedures should be allowed to do so, and whether children born will enjoy a proper and sound family life. Yet it is argued that the love and devotion with which they would be reared and brought up would greatly mitigate such adverse effects. Antisocial behaviour can be readily evolved in those children naturally conceived.

Ethical concerns have been raised on a number of other issues, including:

1. The risk of abnormalities, or subsequent miscarriages, as a result of the manipulation of the gametes, that is the sperm and the egg. While there is no evidence of an increase in congenital abnormalities in babies conceived by means of IVF the number of babies born are too few for statistical proof to be forthcoming to date. Embryos fertilized *in vitro* were replaced in the uteri of 1200 women between October 1980 and April 1983. Of this number, although there have been three pregnancies which ended in abortion producing defective fetuses, only one child born has had an abnormality — a cardiac aberration in one of the twins born in Melbourne, Australia.[28]

The Report of the RCOG Ethics Committee (1983) concludes that the proportion of abnormalities following IVF is therefore no higher than would occur under 'natural' circumstances. At a Dublin Congress on infertility and sterility, Steptoe and Edwards (1983) predicted that IVF might soon be even more efficient than mother nature, producing more babies with fewer abnormalities.

The question of fetal abnormality is still one that has to be borne in mind, however, for as yet until more data are available to compare with the rate of abnormalities in spontaneous abortions and natural births, no one can say definitely whether IVF leads to any increase in abnormal fetuses.[29]

2. Spare embryos: What happens when more than a single egg is obtained from a woman and fertilized in the laboratory? If only one or two embryos are implanted in the woman's uterus what happens to the others? There are three alternatives. They can be (a) discarded, (b) used for experimental purposes (see p.195), or (c) preserved for future use (see p.180). Each of these options is controversial, for each raises the issues of the legal and social status of the early human embryo.

Those who believe that human life begins at conception would find the disposal of such embryos deeply disturbing for it would amount to an act of abortion. It is a well known fact, however, that a large number of human embryos *in vivo* are expelled from the bodies of pregnant women as a result of natural processes. About one third are terminated naturally within the first three months of pregnancy, and a high proportion of fetuses lost in this way are genetically abnormal. One might say, therefore, that this is nature's way of eliminating genetic mistakes. A distinction should be made between ova which become fertilized but do not implant and cannot develop further even if the cells are still alive, and those in which implantation occurs and therefore the route for nourishment and development is available.

Such a high rate of embryonic loss often occurs in the first two weeks of life, even before the woman believes she is pregnant. A couple who are attempting to conceive a child normally accept such embryonic wastage as the perfectly acceptable price to be paid for the birth of a healthy child.

There are those who would see such embryonic discard as providing no moral justification for any *intentional* replication for any reason whatsoever, and regard the status of the embryo as to some degree different from that of the fetus. Married couples who engage in sexual relations, they argue, do not intend the embryo discards which may in fact occur. They are not *'causing'* abortions. The natural loss of embryos in early pregnancy does not in itself provide a 'go-ahead' for deliberately aborting them, any more than still births give justification for new born infanticide.

Attempts to define the moral status of the embryo are sometimes made by asking the question, When does life begin?, which is at the heart of the ongoing abortion debate. Such an undeniably difficult question produces widely different responses, if what is sought is 'a subsequent and specific time-related answer'. There are a number of possibilities —

conception, implantation, ensoulment, quickening, birth. There seem no neat and tidy conclusions and a clear-cut answer is extremely difficult. If 'conception' is considered, certain further questions have to be asked. Do we assign a special value to the conceptus at this time? If so, are we morally obliged to conserve the life of a newly fertilized ovum as we are the twenty-eight week fetus or the new born child? What about the wastefulness of human life given the natural prevalence of early miscarriages? Can the 'moment' of conception be considered as a single and definite event in time?

Should there be a duty to respect the absolute inviolability of the embryo because it is human, our present methods of contraception would have to be reconsidered and the use of the intra-uterine device (IUCD) — the coil — defended. There are at present fifty million users of IUCD, which is a device which prevents implantation of the human embryo in the uterus and allows it to be rejected. It cannot be morally worse to end the life of an embryo *in vitro* than it is to do so *in vivo*.[30]

Traditional Roman Catholic theology held that the human soul is present from the 'moment' of conception (Tertullian: 'immediate animation'). Another school believed the soul or 'animus' entered after conception, probably in the second trimester (Aristotle, Augustine, Aquinas: 'delayed animation'). Some modern theologians consider this particular doctrine uncertain and place it in positive doubt. Reasons given for these reservations are the possibilities of twinning and recombination, and the loss of a large number of fertilized human embryos.

There appears to be no factual evidence to settle the question, When does life begin? The view which seems to be adopted by most people is that of a 'sliding scale' of fetal value, that as the fetus develops in the uterus so its intrinsic value increases. As its physical development progresses so its destruction becomes more and more difficult to justify. The fertilized ovum gains rights and safeguards as it develops, so that above twenty weeks abortion should only be allowed for serious reasons. Human life is continual and it is not a question of beginning or ending at any one definitive stage or place. In human reproduction life never begins — it is only passed on by means of conception. We simply cannot speak of the 'moment' when life 'occurs'.

In an attempt to analyse the riddle Grobstein (1982) has proposed six statements which, he believes, are scientifically valid and accepted as such by most scientists:

1. Life is continuous from generation to generation. It does not arise anew in each individual. Life does not, therefore, begin at fertilization.
2. Human life is no exception.
3. Fertilization does, however, mark two important stages in the continuity of life. It is at this point that the egg becomes active and that the genetic individuality of the embryo is established by the combination of genes from both of the parents.
4. The one-celled embryo, or zygote, is, however, not a new individual. By common standards it has none of the characteristics we associate with people. By scientific standards, the zygote is not an individual because it may split to form two individuals (twins) even two weeks after fertilization and, at least in mice, scientists can join two early embryos to form a single individual.
5. In the very early stages, scientists can remove cells from a mouse embryo, without affecting the outcome of the development. The cells in early embryos are not specialized parts of a multicellular organism.
6. Only after several days of development is it possible to distinguish between cells that will form the embryo and those that will form the placenta.

He affirms that at the cellular or genetic level human life exists before, during and after fertilization. But the emergence of a multi-cellular individual (with a unique set of genes) occurs only two weeks after fertilization.[31]

Whichever stage is chosen, difficulties arise, and as the RCOG Report (1983) concludes, the proper moral and by far the more helpful question to pose is not, When does life begin?, but rather, At what point in the development of the embryo do we attribute to it the protection due to a human being? Knowing that in the natural process large numbers of fertilized ova are lost before implantation, the Royal College suggests it is morally unconvincing to claim inviolability for an organism with which nature is so prodigal.

THE EARLY DEVELOPMENT OF THE HUMAN EMBRYO IN VITRO

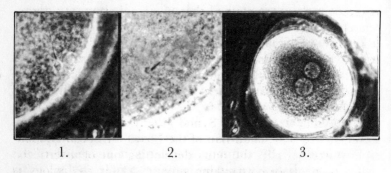

1.   2.   3.

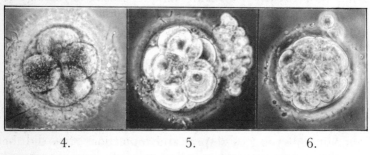

4.   5.   6.

1. The sperm approaching the ovum.
2. The sperm penetrating the cell membrane.
3. The fertilized ovum at the 2-cell stage.
4. The 4-cell stage.
5. The cells of the embryo divide to form the 8-cell and 16 cell stages (6).

(The author is most grateful to Dr Robert Edwards for providing these slides for publication.)

What then is the moral status of a human zygote (a fertilized human embryo)? How are we to regard it? It is clearly alive for it grows and divides. Although it is not yet organized into distinctive parts or organs, the blastocyst is an organic whole, self-developing, and genetically unique. It is human insofar as it belongs to the human species, homo sapiens, and has an individuality in the sense that it has all the genetic material to make a mature human being if all goes well. Yet it is barely visible to the naked eye, and shows no human characteristics whatsoever when observed under a micro-scope. (When I viewed a fertilized human embryo under the microscope it was explained that its actual size was approx-imately that of 'a full stop'.) It appears as a cluster of cells, but it is at least potential humanity, and its small size has, of course, little relation to any judgement of its 'humanness'. As such it should elicit our feelings of awe and respect, but not necessarily to the same extent as those given to a fully devel-oped human being.

Addressing the General Synod (1976), the then Bishop of London, who was Chairman of the Board for Social Respon-sibility, stated that 'the fetus developing out of a fertilized ovum is, genetically speaking unique; as far as biology is concerned, the full potential for human personality is present from the time of fertilization. But it is equally clear that the fullness of what we understand by 'a person' is not present from conception onwards; a person's capacity to know him-self, to relate to others and notably to respond to God grows with his growth in time and space, and of course continues to the end of his life'.[32] If such a viewpoint is accepted the fertilized embryo is seen as not yet a person but potential humanity deserving of respect and protection. How did the Dean of Durham view the moral status of the human embryo?

> 'It is an individual, because it has a unique complement of genes which stamps on it its individuality and will continue to do so if it is allowed to develop. It already has the plan, physically speaking, of its own future develop-ment, but it does not yet have any intelligent or even sensitive characteristics: it is "on the way" to them. I don't think that the fact of its being an individual necess-arily implies that we ought to give it the same protection as we should give an adult human being. I don't think you should give it that until there is some kind of cerebral activity, and that depends on brain formation."

Did he think it had sentience?

> 'It hasn't any sentience. Sentience is important because it is a ground for giving certain protection. It is morally wrong to cause sentient beings pain or suffering which is not otherwise justified. So I should not be prepared to cause the embryo pain or suffering, but I'm not sure at the moment that I should wish to give it the full protection which we give to human beings, including unborn human beings just before birth.'

Would there be justification in allowing spare embryos just to be left?

> 'I think it would be morally justifiable to let them die. This often happens naturally after fertilization, since a large percentage of fertilized ova never implant. On the other hand, I should be worried if embryos were used for any old experiment.'

The Archbishop of York saw the moral status of the embryo as

> 'a bundle of potentialities which are, and will remain, mere potentialities unless a great deal more happens, of which the first step is implantation. It is, in my view, absurd to talk about a fertilized ovum as if it were in some sense already a human person.'

Dealing with the question as to when the embryo should receive the same ethical safeguards and protection as an adult, he considered that

> 'whatever we might say to the contrary, I suspect that we do not give a fetus the same ethical consideration we would give to an adult until quite late in pregnancy, and the fact that we do not is shown quite clearly by the normal reactions to miscarriages. These may be tragic, but nothing like as tragic as the death of a child.'

As regards many of the ethical issues involved in IVF, greater attention is to be devoted to possible future developments and applications of the techniques, rather than to what at present is being carried out solely to alleviate some of the problems involved in infertility. The most significant of the new ethical problems initiated by the procedures of IVF is that of experimentation on human embryos.

1. Experimentation: The ethical questions of research and possible disposal centre to a great extent on the status of the early embryo and its rights, and on the balance between the opportunities for good and the values of life. If the embryo is deserving of respect it is difficult to justify creating it solely for the purpose of experimentation. Many would see such experimentation as an offence against the sanctity of human life. This was very much in the mind of Professor Ian Kennedy when I talked to him about the moral status of the human embryo, and what respect, if any, should be accorded it:

> 'We are speaking about what respect is due to an entity whether fertilized egg, blastocyst or embryo. The respect due to it may be determined by what status we attribute to it. If it were a stone or a vegetable it would command little or no respect. If it is like you or me — deemed to be like you or me — it demands the respect that we give to human life. We would have to find very strong reasons for neglecting it. The only way that I can resolve this is to suggest that the entity ought to be regarded as in reality what it is — a growing thing which, as it physically acquires characteristics, in my view, morally calls for greater respect. There is, as it were, a progression, the respect following and increasing with that physiological development which is causing it to become more and more like us. Then, I think you have to ask at what stage along this process you regard the embryo as warranting respect as human life. It could be, for example, when it develops those physiological capacities which allow it to be a sentient, that is the development of the central nervous system during the process of organogenesis. Before reaching that stage some may argue that we can, perhaps, do experiments on it, if it happens to be scientifically worthwhile. When it has acquired the characteristics which I consider and describe as a human, then, obviously, one would have great difficulty in justifying doing these things to it. Having decided that at some

point it has a claim to respect, I can at the same time be reconciled to its destruction if there is a conflict between the claims of it and the claims of the mother as in the case of abortion.'

On the basis of his view about the acquisition of human qualities, he felt:

'it would be perfectly legitimate to carry out experimentation on these four, eight, sixteen cell embryos, indeed to carry out experimentation on the embryo up until about the period at which it reaches that stage during organogenesis at which it acquires those features that mark it out as a human being. But I still have objections to experimentation on embryos of this tiny size. These objections do not turn upon the status of the embryo but on the intention of the investigator. If the intention was to create a surplus number of embryos just for the purpose of experimenting then I have a slightly difficult problem. The intention to me is crucial. Although I am still admitting that the embryo does not have that status whereby it is entitled to respect as a human being, nonetheless I have a strong objection to creating something potentially human just for the purpose of experimenting on it. That is going beyond where I myself feel comfortable morally.'

It is important, however, to make a clear distinction between 'research' and 'therapy'. Research which is scientifically sound might enable valuable information to be obtained about the process of reproduction relative to clinical problems such as contraception, the treatment of infertility and inherited diseases, and how genetic defects arise and are transmitted. Our genetic make-up is determined at the very time of fertilization. Each year about two per cent of all babies are born with defects which have a genetic basis, as distinct from birth defects brought about by such factors as drugs, excessive alcohol, and smoking habits of the mother. Some of the misery and consequences of those so affected, as well as those who care for them, are immeasurable.

Some of the doctors who are working in the field of *in vitro* fertilization already keep spare embryos alive for several days in order to observe how they grow and behave. Scientists at the Centre for Reproductive Biology in Edinburgh in their research are at present using embryos which have been created from the ova of women who have had surgery on their ovaries. The embryos are fixed in alcohol when they have reached the egg cell stage at the end of approximately three days. The object of such examinations and observations is to explore the number and arrangements of the particles of genetic material known as the chromosomes which are inside the cells. As a result of such study it is hoped to reveal some of the fundamental causes of genetic defects and abnormalities.

There are a number of researchers who would wish to take experimentation further. They would like to keep the embryo alive for up to a period of six weeks to see the cells multiply and articulate into different parts of the body. During this stage in embryonic development are to be observed the early formation of the brain, the limbs, the spinal cord, and the heart. Scientists state that work on live embryos during this period would enable them to combat other embryos developing into malformed babies, and so help eliminate such a common genetic defect as spina bifida which appears in the third week of the embryo's life.

A number of these developments, none of which has yet taken place, are commonly identified more sensationally with the term 'genetic engineering'. In 'gene therapy' embryos would be examined for chromosomal abnormalities, and would either be discarded or repaired. In Britain serious single gene defects (cystic fibrosis, muscular dystrophy and haemophilia are the most common) affect just under one per cent of children. Discussing the ethics of such therapy Williamson (1982) emphasizes two clear starting points, both of which he considers to be fundamental to most humanistic and religious views. 'The first is that any person whether well or ill, deserves respect as an individual. Patients, however ill they may be, cannot be used as laboratory animals . . . the second underlying ethical rule is, that the medical profession should do all it can to prevent serious handicap.'[33]

Useful and promising as such possibilities of research appear to be, the basic question is, how far is it morally permissible to go in human embryonic research in the interests of combating disease? The codes that govern experimentation on human adults (see p.12) state that such experiments should not take place if there is a danger they would suffer permanent injury or death in the process. To what extent should such principles apply to human embryos? On the question of 'informed consent', the MRC (Medical Research Council) in its statement on *Research related to Human Fertilization and Embryology* (1983), asserts that informed consent to research involving human ova or sperm should be obtained in every case from the donor(s); sperm from sperm banks should not be used unless collected and preserved specifically for a research purpose. Approval for each experiment should be obtained from the appropriate scientific and local ethical committees. The statement also outlines that the aim of the research should be clearly defined and directly relevant to clinical problems, such as contraception or the differential diagnosis and treatment of infertility and inherited diseases.[34]

I discussed the problem of research on human embryos with two of the leading authorities in the field of *in vitro* fertilization. Both saw it as a contentious subject. Dr Robert Edwards emphasized the enormous potential for good in studying early embryos:

> 'Identifying those with genetic defects, studying differentiation and normal and abnormal growth, teratogenesis, aspects of cancer, even the use of embryonic stem cells in medicine — the list is almost endless. The enormous research potential for science and medicine, and consequent benefits for ameliorating mental and physical suffering, is for me decisive in debates on the ethical dilemma. A conflict arises for many of us contemplating these research studies. Decisions about research are made easily by those who believe the embryo has no rights at all, but not by those with reservations.'*

*Dr R. G. Edwards further develops these viewpoints in his Galton Lecture 1982. (See *Developments in Human Reproduction and their Eugenic, Ethical Implications*. Proceedings from the Nineteenth Annual Symposium of the Eugenics Society, London, 1982. Ed Carter, C.O., Academic Press, London, 1983, pp. 53–115.)

Professor Ian Craft also pointed to some of the advantages of research in eliminating and preventing abnormalities and disease:

> 'On the one hand some feel that the human embryo has such sanctity that nothing should be done to it; on the other hand some would consider that we have a duty to observe and evaluate early stages of human development so that it might be possible to eliminate and prevent abnormalities and disease. If you are to consider just the problem of infertility it is pertinent that we have very little information about what nutritional requirements are necessary for an early human embryo, and you will appreciate that there could be advantages for those seeking *in vitro* fertilization if research in this context was undertaken, since it might lead to development of a better culture medium which could maximize chances of optimum embryo development and successful implantation. My personal opinion is that we should develop the latter approach, since we have an onus as clinicians to prevent undue distress if at all possible and improvement in our success rates are directed towards these ends.'

The late Report, *Choices in Childlessness*, (1982) drew attention to some of the problems arising from experiments in the sphere of *in vitro* fertilization and reached the conclusion that some experiments on 'spare' embryos might be morally justifiable, but not all. The Report recommended that 'society needs encouragement to think through the moral and legal implications of these procedures *now*, and to take whatever steps are considered necessary to prevent unethical and undesirable developments'. The working party's chairman, Dr Peter Baelz, Dean of Durham, and former Professor of Moral and Pastoral Theology at Oxford, commenting on recent developments in the field of *in vitro* experimentation cautioned that 'the kind of language we use is important, because it is these terms which fix our own moral reactions. There are some experiments you might do with fertilized ova which don't necessarily count as experiments with *babies* in test-tubes. There has to be a careful look into the types of experiment possible.' (*Church Times*, October 1982). The Chief Rabbi (Sir

Immanuel Jakobovits) in his evidence to the Warnock Commission gave as his opinion that research on fertilization *in vitro* was legitimate if it was to cure infertility or correct abnormalities in a fetus.

The Roman Catholic Church sees experimentation on human embryos as morally wrong, for it considers that embryos are human beings from the first moment of their existence. Its teaching asserts that 'such new life is the life not of a potential human being but of a human being with potential'.[35]

Others challenge the view that the human embryo has such 'rights' of a human being from fertilization. The MRC suggests that the embryo is not entitled to the 'rights' of humans until it has implanted. There are those who would see such 'rights' only acceptable when the embryo reaches the stage of a being who can feel, when its brain develops in the normal course of pregnancy (i.e. a number of days after the end of the implantation process). The Royal College of Obstetricians and Gynaecologists is of the opinion that the human embryo assumes human status when it starts to have a brain, and maintains that experimentation should stop as soon as the first cells destined to form part of the brain appear (i.e. the seventeenth day of its existence). Some researchers argue that experimentation should be permitted until the first signs of electrical activity in the brain, which would be about the forty-second day in the life of the embryo. Once the embryo has the status of being human it should definitely not be a subject of experimentation.

Experiments that are to be carried out must have scientific value and it is of the utmost importance that no suffering is inflicted nor, indeed, death, by means of experimentation on any sentient being. A definite line has to be drawn somewhere, and at that point experiments must stop. Unless this is so all sorts of horrifying implications might possibly follow. Such is the speed of scientific advance it seems that the earlier the line is drawn the better.

2. *Cloning:* Although not a practical proposition at present there are those who see that cloning reproduction might have medical and social advantages — members would be all ident-

ical forms and so make possible the free exchange of organ transplants with no concern for graft rejection. But for this to be achieved the 'cloned' babies would have to be grown to a size large enough for the organs to be removed and transplanted. At this stage the fetus would already possess all its human characteristics. Procedures of this nature raise the most formidable ethical issues.

Again others would see cloning being employed to permit women who cannot produce an egg cell, or men who cannot produce sperm, donating one of their body cell nuclei for introduction into a donated egg, and so contributing to the production of children. Fletcher (1974) predicted that cloning might be necessary to produce pairs or teams of people for specialized tasks in the community — astronauts, deep-sea divers, surgical groups.[36]

One of the major ethical concerns centres on the problem of possible laboratory mistakes during the process of cloning. Ramsey (1975) cautions about the possibility of subhuman or para-human individuals being produced, as well as 'clonal farming', offering everyone who could afford it a supply of 'identical twin' organs whenever a transplant was needed. Both Ramsey and Habgood (1980) also stress how cloning would threaten to undermine the human and personal elements in parenthood, as well as the loss of the unique existence and importance each of us has, from the christian point of view, 'because we stand, whether we know it or not, in a unique relationship with God'.[37]

Conclusions

The highest standard of scientific skill and ethical concern are to be applied by all who work or study in this sphere of extra-corporeal fertilization. In his Horizon Lecture (1983) Dr R. G. Edwards stated: 'One definite attitude we must never abandon is the search for scientific truth in relation to ethics. All our knowledge about fertilization, about human embryology, must be scrutinized closely and understood, because any ethical standard must acknowledge truth, or observed fact. Any other standard is misleading, and is bound to lead to error. We must also demonstrate our ethics of care to the embryos placed temporarily in our custody, by applying the greatest skills and highest standards in our clinics.'

In attempting to consider such complex problems in the light of the Christian faith there can be no room for ready-made solutions nor hasty moral judgements, whether of condemnation or approval. It would surely be wrong to adopt a negative stand or out-of-hand rejection of some of these advances in human knowledge merely on the grounds of their innovation and sophistication; neither should they be abandoned because of the possibility of abuse or of future possibilities. Rather is it the duty of the christian to examine them in the light of God's revealed purpose.

The fact that we can do something does not necessarily mean that we ought to do it. The recent Report, *Choices in Childlessness*, (1982) does well to remind us that 'technological power does not guarantee truly human solutions to the deepest human problems. Cleverness is not the same thing as wisdom. The question where to place lines, where to draw the line, remains as important as ever'.[38]

The extensions of newly acquired knowledge and the power in the whole field of human fertilization and embryology, together with the responsibilities and opportunities which they present, are to be seen as a part of, rather than a challenge to, God's ordering of his world. It is up to man to see that he does not abuse them nor deliberately use them for evil ends. Grobstein (1982) rightly emphasizes the need for prudence as well as for vision. 'For example, many would be reassured to know that the intent of any intervention in human reproduction would be to benefit individuals and not to "improve" the species as a whole. Though these two are linked, in contemporary thinking the first is generally understood and accepted, the second is burdened by suspicion and fraught with uncertainties as to how "improvement" will be defined — and by whom. It would also be reassuring to know that defects that *limit* self-realization are the legitimate target; that conservation and fuller fruition of humanity as we know it is the goal, not the "engineering" of new forms of human life.'[39]

The greatest of care and judgement is needed to scrutinize closely and evaluate diligently the contributions which these medical and scientific techniques may bring to a truly human life, and to reassure against over-enthusiasm and irresponsibility. Modern technology is advancing so speedily that it is becoming more and more imperative to examine some of its ethical, social and legal implications *now* so that scientific action does not outstrip the moral principles on which it should be founded. Such a challenge concerns us all.

The author wishes to acknowledge his gratitude to Bryan Hibbard, Professor of Obstetrics, Welsh National School of Medicine, Cardiff, for commenting upon and reading through the original draft of this chapter for medical accuracy.

* * * * *

The Warnock Report

The Committee of Inquiry into Human Fertilization and Embryology, which was established by the Government in July 1982, and chaired by Dame Mary Warnock, presented its Report in June 1984. Among its main recommendations are the following:

Licensing Body and its functions:
The establishment of a new statutory licensing authority to regulate both research and those infertility services which are recommended to be subject to control (13.3).

All practitioners offering such services should only be provided under license, and all premises used for infertility services to be licensed by the Licensing Body (13.7).

Techniques for the alleviation of infertility:
AID should be available on a properly organized basis and subject to the licensing arrangements of above Body (4.16).

IVF to continue to be available subject to licensing and inspection (5.10).

Egg donation to be accepted as a recognized technique in the treatment of infertility (6.6).

Embryo donation involving donated semen and egg which are brought together *in vitro* be accepted (7.4).

Donated embryos and gametes to be offered to those at risk of transmitting hereditary disorders (9.3).

The use of frozen eggs in therapeutic procedures should not be undertaken until research has shown that no unacceptable risk is involved; the clinical use of frozen embryos may continue to be developed. All above procedures to be under review of the Licensing Body (10.2).(10.3)

A maximum of ten years for storage of embryos after which time the storage authority should be responsible for their use or disposal (bearing in mind any previously expressed wishes in relation to disposal) (10.10).

Principles of Provision:
Counselling should be available to all infertile couples and third parties at any stage of treatment both in private sector and NHS provision (3.4).

A formal consent in writing by both partners should always be obtained before treatment begins (4.23).

A gradual move towards a system where semen donors should be given only their expenses (4.27).

A limit of ten children who can be fathered by one donor (4.26).

Legal limits on Research:
The human embryo to be afforded protection in law (11.17).

Research conducted on human *in vitro* embryos and the handling of such embryos should be permitted only under licence (11.18).

No live human embryo derived from *in vitro* fertilization, whether frozen or unfrozen, may be kept alive, if not transferred to a women, beyond fourteen days after fertilization, nor may it be used as a research subject after that time. The handling or using of any live human embryo as a research subject beyond that limit to be a criminal offence (11.22).

No research should be carried out on a spare embryo without the informed consent of the couple from whom the embryo was generated. (11.24).

Legal Changes:
The AID child should in law be treated as the legitimate child of its mother and her husband where they have both consented to the treatment (4.17).

The law should be changed so as to permit the husband to be registered as the father, (subject to 4.17). If desired the father's name may be followed in the birth register by the words 'by donation' (4.25).

The child, on reaching the age of eighteen, should have access to basic information about the donor's ethnic origin and genetic health, and legislation be enacted to provide the right of access to this (4.21).

When a child is born to a woman following egg donation the mother giving birth should, for all purposes, be regarded in law as the mother of that child, and the egg donor have no rights or obligations in respect of the child. If desired the mother's name may be followed in the birth register by the words 'by donation' (6.8). The same legislation should cover children born as a result of embryo donation (7.6).

Provision by statute that all surrogacy agreements are illegal contracts and unenforceable in the courts (8.19).

The creation or operation of agencies in the United Kingdom whose purposes include the recruitment of women for surrogate pregnancy, or making arrangements for individuals or couples who wish to utilize the services of a carrying mother to be a criminal offence (8.18).

Report of the Committee of Inquiry into Human Fertilization and Embryology H.M.S.O. 1984.

Appendix I

(a) The Nuremberg Code (1947)

On August 19, 1947, a war crimes tribunal at Nuremberg rendered judgment on 23 German defendants, mostly physicians, who were accused of crimes involving experiments on human subjects. The judgment laid down ten standards to which physicians must conform when carrying out experiments on human subjects, as follows:

PERMISSIBLE MEDICAL EXPERIMENTS 'The great weight of the evidence before us is to the effect that certain types of medical experiments on human beings, when kept within reasonably well-defined bounds, conform to the ethics of the medical profession generally. The protagonists of the practice of human experimentation justify their views on the basis that such experiments yield results for the good of society that are unprocurable by other methods or means of study. All agree, however, that certain basic principles must be observed in order to satisfy moral, ethical and legal concepts:

1. The voluntary consent of the human subject is absolutely essential. This means that the person involved should have legal capacity to give consent; should be so situated as to be able to exercise free power of choice, without the intervention of any element of force, fraud, deceit, duress, overreaching, or other ulterior form of constraint of coercion; and should have sufficient knowledge and comprehension of the elements of the subject matter involved as to enable him to make an understanding and enlightened decision. This latter element requires that before the acceptance of an affirmative decision by the experimental subject there should be made known to him the nature, duration, and purpose of the experiment; the method and means by which it is to be conducted; all inconveniences and hazards reasonably to be expected; and the effects upon his health or person which may possibly come from his participation in the experiment.

The duty and responsibility for ascertaining the quality of the consent rests upon each individual who initiates, directs, or engages in the experiment. It is a personal duty and responsibility which may not be delegated to another with impunity.

2. The experiment should be such as to yield fruitful results for the good of society, unprocurable by other methods or means of study, and not random and unnecessary in nature.

3. The experiment should be so designed and based on the results of animal experimentation and a knowledge of the natural history of the disease or other problem under study that the anticipated results justify the performance of the experiment.

4. The experiment should be so conducted as to avoid all unnecessary physical and mental suffering and injury.

5. No experiment should be conducted where there is an *a priori* reason to believe that death or disabling injury will occur; except, perhaps, in those experiments where the experimental physicians also serve as subjects.

6. The degree of risk to be taken should never exceed that determined by the humanitarian importance of the problem to be solved by the experiment.

7. Proper preparations should be made and adequate facilities provided to protect the experimental subject against even remote possibilities of injury, disability, or death.

8. The experiment should be conducted only by scientifically qualified persons. The highest degree of skill and care should be required through all stages of the experiment of those who conduct or engage in the experiment.

9. During the course of the experiment the human subject should be at liberty to bring the experiment to an end if he has reached the physical or mental state where continuation of the experiment seems to him to be impossible.

10. During the course of the experiment the scientist in charge must be prepared to terminate the experiment at any stage, if he has probable cause to believe, in the exercise of the good faith, superior skill, and careful judgment required of him, that a continuation of the experiment is likely to result in injury, disability, or death to the experimental subject.

(b) **Declaration of Helsinki (1964)**
RECOMMENDATIONS GUIDING DOCTORS IN CLINICAL RESEARCH

Introduction

It is the mission of the doctor to safeguard the health of the people. His knowledge and conscience are dedicated to the fulfilment of this mission.

The Declaration of Geneva of The World Medical Association binds the doctor with the words: 'The health of my patient will be my first consideration'; and the International Code of Medical Ethics declares that 'Any act or advice which could weaken physical or mental resistance of a human being may be used only in his interest.'

Because it is essential that the results of laboratory experiments be applied to human beings to further scientific knowledge and to help suffering humanity, the World Medical Association has prepared the following recommendations as a guide to each doctor in clinical research. It must be stressed that the standards as drafted are only a guide to physicians all over the world. Doctors are not relieved from criminal, civil and ethical responsibilities under the laws of their own countries.

In the field of clinical research a fundamental distinction must be recognized between clinical research in which the aim is essentially therapeutic for a patient, and the clinical research, the essential object of which is purely scientific and without therapeutic value to the person subjected to the research.

I Basic Principles

1. Clinical research must conform to the moral and scientific principles that justify medical research and should be based on laboratory and animal experiments or other scientifically established facts.

2. Clinical research should be conducted only by scientifically qualified persons and under the supervision of a qualified medical man.

3. Clinical research cannot legitimately be carried out unless the importance of the objective is in proportion to the inherent risk to the subject.

4. Every clinical research project should be preceded by careful assessment of inherent risks in comparison to foreseeable benefits to the subject or to others.

5. Special caution should be exercised by the doctor in performing clinical research in which the personality of the subject is liable to be altered by drugs or experimental procedures.

II Clinical Research Combined with Professional Care

1. In the treatment of the sick person, the doctor must be free to use a new therapeutic measure, if in his judgement it offers hope of saving life, re-establishing health, or alleviating suffering.

If at all possible, consistent with patient psychology, the doctor should obtain the patient's freely given consent after the patient has been given a full explanation. In case of legal incapacity, consent should also be procured from the legal guardian; in case of physical incapacity the permission of the legal guardian replaces that of the patient.

2. The doctor can combine clinical research with professional care, the objective being the acquisition of new medical knowledge, only to the extent that clinical research is justified by its therapeutic value for the patient.

III Non-Therapeutic Clinical Research

1. In the purely scientific application of clinical research carried out on a human being, it is the duty of the doctor to remain the protector of the life and health of that person on whom clinical research is being carried out.

2. The nature, the purpose and the risk of clinical research must be explained to the subject by the doctor.

3(a) Clinical research on a human being cannot be undertaken without his free consent after he has been informed; if he is legally incompetent, the consent of the legal guardian should be procured.

3(b) The subject of clinical research should be in such a mental, physical and legal state as to be able to exercise fully his power of choice.

3(c) Consent should as a rule be obtained in writing. However, the responsibility for clinical research always remains with the research worker; it never falls on the subject even after consent is obtained.

4(a) The investigator must respect the right of each individual to safeguard his personal integrity, especially if the subject is in a dependent relationship to the investigator.

4(b) At any time during the course of clinical research the subject or his guardian should be free to withdraw permission for research to be continued.

The investigator or the investigating team should discontinue the research if in his or their judgement it may, if continued, be harmful to the individual.

Appendix II

The Human Tissue Act 1961

An Act to make provision with respect to the use of parts of bodies of deceased persons for therapeutic purposes and purposes of medical education and research and with respect to the circumstances in which post-mortem examinations may be carried out; and to permit the cremation of bodies removed for anatomical examination.

[27th July, 1961]

Be it enacted by the Queen's most Excellent Majesty, by and with the advice and consent of the Lords Spiritual and Temporal, and Commons, in this present Parliament assembled, and by the authority of the same, as follows:-

1.–(1) If any person, either in writing at any time or orally in the presence of two or more witnesses during his last illness, has expressed a request that his body or any specified part of his body be used after his death for therapeutic purposes or for purposes of medical education or research, the person lawfully in possession of his body after his death may, unless he has reason to believe that the request was subsequently withdrawn, authorise the removal from the body of any part or, as the case may be, the specified part, for use in accordance with the request.

Removal of parts of bodies for medical purposes.

(2) Without prejudice to the foregoing subsection, the person lawfully in possession of the body of a deceased person may authorise the removal of any part from the body for use for the said purposes if, having made such reasonable enquiry as may be practicable, he has no reason to believe—

(a) that the deceased had expressed an objection to his body being so dealt with after his death, and had not withdrawn it; or

(b) that the surviving spouse or any surviving

relative of the deceased objects to the body being so dealt with.

(3) Subject to subsections (4) and (5) of this section, the removal and use of any part of a body in accordance with an authority given pursuance of this section shall be lawful.

(4) No such removal shall be effected except by a fully registered medical practitioner, who must have satisfied himself by personal examination of the body that life is extinct.

(5) Where a person has reason to believe that an inquest may be required to be held on any body or that a post-mortem examination of the body may be required by the coroner, he shall not, except with the consent of the coroner,—

  (a) give an authority under this section in respect of the body; or
  (b) act on such an authority given by any other person.

(6) No authority shall be given under this section in respect of any body by a person entrusted with the body for the purpose only of its interment or cremation.

(7) In the case of a body lying in a hospital, nursing home or other institution, any authority under this section may be given on behalf of the person having the control and management thereof by any officer or person designated for that purpose by the first-mentioned person.

(8) Nothing in this section shall be construed as rendering unlawful any dealing with, or with any part of, the body of a deceased person which is lawful apart from this Act.

(9) In the application of this section to Scotland, for subsection (5) there shall be substituted the following subsection:-

  "(5) Nothing in this section shall authorise the removal of any part from a body in any case where the procurator fiscal has objected to such removal."

2.–(1) Without prejudice to section fifteen of the Anatomy Act, 1832 (which prevents that Act from being construed as applying to post-mortem examinations directed to be made by a competent legal authority), that Act shall not be construed as applying to any post-mortem examination carried out for the purpose of establishing or confirming the causes of death or of investigating the existence or nature of abnormal conditions.

(2) No postmortem examination shall be carried out otherwise than by or in accordance with the instructions of a fully registered medical practitioner, and no post-mortem examination which is not directed or requested by the coroner or any other competent legal authority shall be carried out without the authority of the person lawfully in possession of the body; and subsections (2), (5), (6) and (7) of section one of this Act shall, with the necessary modifications, apply with respect to the giving of that authority.

3. The provision to be made and the certificate to be transmitted under section thirteen of the Anatomy Act, 1832, in respect of a body removed for anatomical examination may, instead of being provision for and cremation of the body in accordance with the Cremation Acts, 1902 and 1952, and a certificate of the cremation.

Cremation of bodies after anatomical examination.

2 Edw. 7. c. 8. 15 & 16 Geo. 6. & 1 Eliz. 2. c. 31.

4.–(1) This Act may be cited as the Human Tissue Act, 1961.

(2) The Corneal Grafting Act, 1952, is hereby repealed.

Short title, etc. 15 & 16 Geo. 6. & 1 Eliz. 2. c. 28.

(3) This Act shall come into operation at the expiration of a period of two months beginning with the day on which it is passed.

(4) This Act does not extend to Northern Ireland.

(Reproduced by permission of the Controller of Her Majesty's Stationery Office).

Appendix III

Questions for Discussion

1. HUMAN EXPERIMENTATION:

(a) Has the patient a sense of duty or responsibility to co-operate in research?

(b) Who is to define ethical and moral rights and obligations of all those involved in human experimentation — medical, paramedical, patients?

(c) Is there a conflict between individual rights and the rights of society? How far can we ask one human being to take part in trials which may not benefit himself, or, perhaps, even the present generation?

(d) How much information must patients be given? Can there ever be such a thing as 'fully informed consent'?

(e) What methodology, if any, should be used in reaching judgements about which research projects are ethical? Who is qualified to review the performance of ethical committees?

(f) Do you consider that 'informed/true consent' is always necessary?

(g) How much flexibility or freedom should investigators be allowed?

(h) Should children be involved in experimentation?

2. ORGAN TRANSPLANTATION:

(a) What do you consider to be some of the factors responsible for the shortage of organs for transplantation?

(b) In the present shortage what do you think should be some of the guidelines used for selection of patients awaiting transplant surgery?

(c) Do you consider that transplant patients (e.g. liver, heart) are being given a meaningful level of life, or a prolonged state of suffering and need?

(d) Within limitations of current financial resources and manpower are transplant operations justifiable?

(e) Are vital organ transplantations justified in terms of results produced?

3. BRAIN-DEATH:

(a) Do you consider the medical criteria for the definition of 'brain death' as outlined in the 1976 and 1979 Royal Colleges' criteria satisfactory?

(b) Is a more specific and objectively stated definition of death necessary for moral and legal purposes?

(c) Is there a case for a statute concerning the occurrence of death which might possibly remove all doubts in the minds of both doctors and public?

(d) Should patients in irreversible coma or suffering from irreparable brain damage, as distinct from 'brain death', be maintained in a 'vegetative state' for an indefinite time?

(e) Is it morally justifiable to prolong such 'life' by artificial means?

4. HANDICAPPED INFANTS — TO SAVE OR LET DIE?:

(a) Who has the 'right' to decide that life with a handicap, even a severe one, is not worth living?

(b) On what ethical principles should the choice be made?

(c) To what extent do you think parents should be involved in decision-making?

(d) How is 'personhood' to be defined?

(e) Is 'sanctity of life' to be an overriding consideration in all incidences? Are heroic efforts to be made to salvage all life?

(f) Who should make these decisions? Doctors? Parents? Committees?

(g) Is withholding treatment ethically different from terminating life? Is there a moral difference between 'killing' and 'letting die', between 'acts' and 'omissions'?

(h) Is society to issue guidelines and if so, which is the most appropriate body to do so?

5. HUMAN FERTILIZATION AND EMBRYOLOGY:

(a) What are some of the harmful psychological and emotional strains and stresses in family relationships which might arise as a consequence of AID?

(b) How far do you consider AID to be a morally justifiable procedure?

(c) (i) Should a donor's wife be informed? (ii) Should the donor be paid? (iii) Should he be accepted if proposed by the sterile couple?

(d) Ought AID children be granted the right to know their real genetic origin?

(e) Since it is now possible to fertilize a human egg *in vitro*, from what moment can the fertilized egg be considered to be an 'individual'? When should it receive the same ethical safeguards and protection as the adult?

(f) Does *in vitro* fertilization fall within the normal perogatives of the practice of medicine in the sense that it is satisfying the desires of human beings rather than practising the art or science of healing?

(g) Is it ethically right to originate a human person completely outside the sexual union of the two spouses?

(h) Is it right to use abortion in order to reduce the incidence of a disease such as Down's syndrome where sufferers are apparently capable of a happy, albeit limited existence?

(i) Should selective abortion be used in the case of all abnormalities identified, or only in the more serious ones?

(j) What are some of the potential long-term implications of the development of 'sperm banks'?

(k) Is there a case for regulation now that freezing of genetic material and cloning are already part of existing procedures?

Glossary

AMNIOCENTESIS
The passage of a needle into the cavity of the womb in order to draw out fluid from the amniotic sac.

ANALGESIC
A remedy that relieves pain.

ANTI-CONVULSANT
A therapeutic agent that prevents or arrests convulsants.

ANTIBIOTIC
Tending to destroy life; designating the extracts of certain organisms employed against infections caused by other organisms.

BARBITURATE
Barbiturates are used in medicine as hypnotic and sedative drugs.

BLASTOCYST
The early embryo consisting of a ball of cells containing a cavity filled with fluid. This stage occurs about five days after fertilization.

CADAVER
A dead body, a corpse.

CATHETER
A hollow tube of metal, glass, hard or soft rubber, rubberized silk, etc. for insertion into a cavity through a narrow canal, for the purpose of discharging the fluid contents of a cavity, or for establishing the patency of a canal.

CEREBRAL CORTEX
The external grey layer of the brain.

CHROMOSOME
Thread-like structures in the cell nucleus that carry the genes; there is generally a constant number for each species.

CLONE
A colony or group of organisms (or an individual organism), or a colony of cells derived from a single organism or cell by asexual reproduction, all having identical characteristics.

COMA
Unconsciousness from which a patient cannot be aroused.

COMATOSE	In a condition of coma.
CONCEPTUS	The developing product of conception throughout pregnancy.
DIAGNOSIS	The art or the act of determining the nature of a disease. The decision reached.
ECTOGENESIS	Growth of a fetus outside of the human body, without the need of the maternal womb.
EGG	The female cell arising in the ovary, when fertilized by a male sperm cell results in an embryo.
ELECTRO-ENCEPHALOGRAM (EEG)	A graphic record of the minute changes in electric potential associated with the activity of the cerebral cortex, as detected by electrodes applied to the surface of the scalp.
EMBRYO	A young organism in the early stage of development. The product of conception up to the third month of pregnancy.
FALLOPIAN TUBE	A uterine tube serving to transport the ovum from the ovary to the exterior.
FETUS	The unborn offspring in the womb from the ninth week until birth.
FOLLICLE (Ovarian)	A small secretory cavity or sac. An ovum and the follicular cells which surround it, lying in the cortex of the ovary.
GAMETE	A male or female reproductive cell capable of entering into union with another in the process of fertilization or of conjugation.
GENE	Any hereditary factor; the ultimate unit in the transmission of hereditary characteristics.
GENETIC	Pertaining to or having reference to origin, mode of production or development. Pertaining to genetics. Produced by genes.
GESTATION	Pregnancy.
HYPOTHERMIA	Subnormal temperature of the body.
INTRACRANIAL HAEMORRHAGE	Haemorrhage within the skull.

MISCARRIAGE	Expulsion of the fetus before it is viable. Abortion.
MYOCARDIAC INFRACTION	Cardiac failure.
NEONATE	A newly born infant.
NEPHROLOGIST	A doctor specializing in the treatment of the kidneys.
NEURAL TUBE DEFECT	Defect of the nerves or nervous tissue of the uterine tube.
NEUROLOGIST	A physician specializing in the diagnosis and treatment of disorders of the nervous system.
NUCLEUS	The structure in the cell that governs cell function.
OBSTETRICIAN	One who practices obstetrics — the branch of medicine that cares for women during pregnancy, labour and the puerperium.
ORTHOPAEDIC	That branch of surgery concerned with corrective treatment of deformities, diseases, and ailments affecting limbs, bones, muscles, joints, etc.
OVARY	One of a pair of glandular organs giving rise to ova, and situated within the pelvic cavity.
PAEDIATRICIAN	A specialist in children's diseases.
PHYSIOTHERAPY	Treatment of disease, injury or deformity by massage, heat, exercises, etc.
PLACEBO	A medicine having no pharmacologic effect.
PLACENTA	The organ on the wall of the uterus to which the embryo is attached by means of the umbilical cord and through which it receives its nourishment. Often referred to as the 'after-birth' because it is delivered soon after the birth of a baby.
PROGNOSIS	A prediction of the duration, course, and termination of a disease, based on all information available in the individual case and knowledge of how the disease behaves generally.

RADIOTHERAPY	The treatment of disease by means of X-rays, radium rays, and other radioactive substances.
RENAL FAILURE	Failure of kidney functioning.
RESUSCITATION	The prevention of asphyxial death by artificial respiration.
SEDATIVE	An agent allaying activity.
SEMEN	The fluid carrying the sperm.
SPERM	The male cells of reproduction.
STILL-BORN	Born dead.
THERAPY	Treatment effecting the cure of disease.
TRAUMA	A wound or injury.
UTERUS	The womb; the hollow female organ of gestation.
VACCINES	Any organism used for preventive inoculation against a specific disease.
VIABLE	Capable of living, applied to a fetus capable of living outside of the uterus.
VIRUS	A general term for the poison of an infectious disease.
ZYGOTE	The early stage of the embryo after fertilization.

References

Chapter 1: Human Experimentation

1. *Small-Pox*, Dixon C. W., J. and A. Churchill, 1962. cf. Sir Edward Mellanby, a former secretary of the Medical Research Council: 'The work . . . of medical men and of nursing staff in controlling disease can only be as good as knowledge allows it to be, and this knowledge has come, and can only come, by medical research.' Mellanby, E., Medical Research in Wartime', *Brit. Med. J.* 1943, 2:352–356.

2. Quoted by Fox, R. C. 'Some social and cultural factors in American society conducive to medical research on human subjects': *Clinical Pharmacology & Therapeutics*, 1960, I: 423–443.

3. *Brit. Med. J.*, 1964, 2:177

4. Ramsey, P., 'The Ethics of a Cottage Industry: Marriage of Community and Research Medicine', *N. Eng. J. Med.* 284, 1971, 700–706. See also: *Medical Matters: The Patient's Consent*, Cook, E. D., Grove Booklet on Ethics. No. 50: 1983.

5. Ingelfinger, F. J., Editorial, *New Eng. J. Med.* 1972, 287: 465–6.

6. Editorial, 'Mind and Cancer', *Lancet*, 1979 1:706–7. Also Fox, B. H., 'Premorbid psychological factors as related to cancer incidence': *J. Behav. Med.* : 1978:1:45–133.
   Loftus, E. F., Fries, J. F., 'Informed Consent may be Hazardous to Health', *Science*, 1979, 204 : 6 April.

7. *J. Med. Ethics*, 1982, 8:59–60.

8. Campbell, A. G. M., 'Infants, Children and Informed Consent', based on inaugural lecture given at University of Aberdeen, *Brit. Med. J.*, 1974, 3:334–338. See also, *The Patient as Person*, Ramsey, P., Newhaven, London, 1970 p. 12.

9. *Lancet*, 1974, 11:398.

10. *Lancet*, 1977, 11:754–5.

11. Dworking, G., 'Legality of consent to nontherapeutic medical research on infants and young children', *Arch. Dis. Child*, 1978, 53:443–446.

12. 'Guidelines to aid ethical committees considering research involving children', Working party on ethics of research in children, *Brit. Med. J.*, 1980, 280:229–31.

13. See McCormick, Richard, A., S. J., 'Proxy Consent in the Experimentation Situation', *Perspectives in Biology and Medicine*, Autumn, 1974.

14. Ramsey, P., *The Patient as Person*, New Haven, London, 1970, p. 14.

15. The BMA *Handbook of Medical Ethics*: 1981.

16. *Dictionary of Medical Ethics* (Revised and Enlarged Edition). Ed. by A. S. Duncan, G. R. Dunstan, R. B. Welbourn, Darton, Longman & Todd, 1981, Art.: 'Clinical trials', Charles F. George: 81–86.

17. For further discussion see: 'Ethics, philosophy and clinical trials', Editorial, *J. Med. Eth.*, 1983, 9:59–60.
    Burkhardt, R., Kienie, G. 'Basic problems in controlled trials'. Ibid 80–84.
    Vere, D. W., 'Problems in controlled trials — a critical response', ibid 85–89.
    Hill, A. B., 'Medical Ethics and Controlled Trials', *Brit. Med. J.*, 1963, 1:1043–1049.
    Lockwood, M. Anscombe, 'Sins of Omission? The non-treatment of controls in clinical trials', The Aristotelian Society, 1983, offprinted from Supplementary Vol LVII, 1983: 207–222.

18. Beecher, H. K. 'Ethics and Clinical Research', *New Eng. J. Med.*, 1966, 274:554–560.
    Pappworth, M. H., *Human Guinea Pigs: Experimentation in Man*, Routledge and Kegan Paul, London 1967.

19. *Brit. Med. J.*, 1981, 282:1010.
    See also: Allen, P., Waters, W. E., 'Attitudes to research ethical committees', *J. Med. Eth.*, 1983, 9:61–65.

20. Whalan, D. J., *Med. J. of Australia*, 1975, 1:491–494.

21. *Ethical issues in experimental medicine in updating life and death*, Ed. Donald E. Cutter, M. H. Pappworth, Boston, Beacon Press, 1969.

22. *Introduction L'Etude de la Médicine Expérimentale*, Paris, Libraire Joseph Gilbert, 1865. pp. 139–140.

Chapter 2: Organ Transplantation

1. Murray, J. E. Merrill, J. P. and Harrison, J. H., 'Renal homotransplantation in identical twins', *Surg. Forum*, 1955, 6:432.

2. Calne, R. Y., *Brit. J. Surg.*, 1961, 48:384.

3. Barnard, C., 'A human Cardiac Transplant: An interim report of a successful operation performed at Groote Schuur Hospital, Cape Town.' *South African J. of Med*, 1967, 41:1271–4.

4. *Cadaveric Organs for Transplantation:* A code of practice including the diagnosis of brain death, drawn up by working party on behalf of the Health Department of Great Britain and Northern Ireland, Oct. 1979, Revised Feb. 1983, 7–8.

5. Jennett, B., *Brit. Med. J.*, 1975, 1 Feb., 252.

6. *UK Transplant Service Review*, 1981: 26.

7. Department of Health and Social Security (1975) Guidance Circular to NHS Authorities: Human Tissue Act HSO (1S)156.

8. Sells, R. A., 'Live Organs from Dead People', *J. Roy. Soc. Med.* 1979, 72: Feb: 112.
   See also Knight, B., 'Forensic Problems in Practice: IV. Law and Ethics in Transplantation', *Practitioner*, 1976, May: 471–4.
   Kennedy, I., 'The Donation and Transplantation of Kidneys: Should the Law be Changed', *J. Med. Eth.*, 1979, 5: 13–21.

9. *Advice from the advisory group on transplantation problems on the question of amending the Human Tissue Act 1961*, MacLennan, H. London, HMSO 1969, CMND 4106, Chaired by Sir Hector MacLennan.

10. Dunstan, G., *Theology*, Vol. LXII, August 1969, 590:339.
    See also Mahoney, J., 'Ethical Aspects of Donor Consent in Transplantation', *J. Med. Eth.*, 1975, 1: 67–70.
    Kennedy, I., Sells, R. A., 'Let's Not Opt Out: Kidney Donation and Transplantation', *J. Med. Eth.*, 1979, 29–32.

11. 'The Shortage of Organs for Clinical Transplantation', *Brit. Med. J.* 1975, 1st Feb., 251–5.

12. For further reference to the problem of selection see Leenen, H. J. J., 'Selection of Patients', *J. Med. Eth.* 1982, 8:33–36.
    Parsons, V. Lock, P., 'Triage and the Patient with Renal Failure', *J. Med. Eth.*, 1980, 6:173–6.
    Parsons, V., 'The Ethical Challenges of Dialysis and Transplantation', *Practitioner*, 1978, 220: 871–7.
    Smith, A., 'Who's to Blame?', *Times Health Supplement*, 1982, Jan 22, 13.
    Kennedy, I., *The Unmasking of Medicine*, Paladin Book, Granada, Revised Ed. 1983, Chapt 7. 181f.
    'Deaths from chronic renal failure under the age of 50', Medical Services Study Group of the Royal College of Physicians, *Brit. Med. J.*, 1981, 283:283–6.
    Knapp, M. S., 'Renal failure — dilemmas and developments', *Brit. Med. J.*, 1982, 284:847–50.
    Fox, R. C., 'Exclusion from Dialysis: Sociologic and Legal Perspective', *Kidney International*, 1981, 19:739–51.

13. Spalak, M., 'Kidney Transplantation — The Hard Sell', *Transplantation Proceedings*, 1982, Vol. XIV. 1, March: 219.

See also Savdie, E., Mahoney, J. F., Caterson, R. J., Stewart, J. H., Etheredge, S. Storey, G., Sheil, A. G. R., 'Long Term Survival after Cadaveric Renal Transplantation', *Brit. Med. J.* 1982, 285: 23 Oct. 1160–3.

14. Calne, R., 'What has happened to Charity?' *Brit. Med. J.* 1982, 284: 3rd April. 998.

15. Spalak, M., 'Kidney Transplantation', *Practitioner*, 1981, 225: July: 987.

16. Parsons, F. M., Ogg, C. S. (Eds) *Renal Failure — Who Cares?*, M. T. P. Press Ltd, International Medical Publications, 1983, 22.

17. *Organ Grafts*, Roy Calne, Edward Arnold, London, 1975.

18. Morris, P. J. Ed. *Tissue Transplantation*, Churchill Livingstone, 1981, 147–60.
    See also Schroeder, J. S. 'Hemodynamic Performance of the Human Transplanted Heart', *Transpl. Proc.*, 1979, 11: 304–8.

19. English, T., Cory-Pearce, R., 'The Current State of Cardiac Transplantation. Papworth Hosp. Cambs', *UK Transplant Service Review*, 1981, 109–119.

20. See Ferriman, A., 'Doctors call for end to heart transplants', *Observer*, 29 August, 1982: 'Hearts in the Right Place', *The Times*, 26 Aug. 1982.
    Draper, P., 'Why Doctors must put their Heart into Prevention', *Guardian*, 12 March 1980.
    cf: 'Cardiac Transplantation: The Second Round', Editorial, *Lancet*, 29 March 1980.
    Hilton, J., 'Heart-swaps help taxpayers', *Sunday Times*, 2 March 1980: 15.

21. Calne, R. Y., 'Orthotopic Liver Grafting in Man', *UK Transplant Service Review*, 1981, 99–108. Also Calne, R. Y., 'Transplant Surgery: Current Status', *Br. J. Surg.*, 1950, 67: 765.
    Calne, R. Y., Williams, R., Lindop, M., Farman, I. V., Tolley, M. E., Rolles, K., MacDougal, E., Neuberger, J., Wyke, R. J., Raftery, A. T., Duffro, T. J., Wight, D. G. P., 'Improved Survival after Orthotopic Liver Grafting', *Brit. Med. J.*, 1981, 283: 11 July.

22. Iglehart, J. K., 'Transplantation: The Problem of Limited Resources', *New Eng. J. Med.*, 1983, 309: 2: 123–8.

23. See also *My Second Chance*, Keith Castle, 1983, Patrick Stephens Ltd, Cambridge.

24. Mahoney, J., 'Ethical Aspects of Donor Consent in Transplantation', *J. Med. Eth.*, 1975, 1: 67.
    cf. Canon G. Bentley, formerly Canon of Windsor: 'The action of the donor seems to me extremely meritorius. It seems to spring from what one might call a "Sermon-on-the-Mount" principle, since it transcends

any ordinary moral system of rights and duties.' *Ethics in Medical Progress: CIBA Foundation Symposium*, Wolsenholme & O'Connor, J. & A. Churchill, 1966.

For further discussion on 'principle of totality' see *Ethics in Medical Progress: CIBA Foundation Symposium*, ibid. 207.

Ramsey, P., *The Patient as Person*, Yale Univ. Press, 6th Printing 1975, 179–81.

25. Jakobovits, I., 'Jewish medical ethics — a brief overview', *J. Med. Eth.*, 1983, 9: 109–112.

26. *A Dictionary of Medical Ethics and Practice*, Thomson, W. A. R., John Wright, Bristol. 1977, 253.

Chapter 3: Brain Death

1. Jennett. B., 'Brain Death 1983', *Practitioner*, 1983, 227:451–4. See also Jennett B., Hessett C., 'Brain Death in Britain as reflected in renal donors'. *Br. Med. J.*, 1981, 283:359.

2. Jennett, B., 'Death, Determination of', Art. *Dictionary of Medical Ethics*, Ed. Duncan, A. S., Dunstan, G. R., Welbourn R. B., Darton, Longman and Todd (Revised and enlarged edition), 1981, 129.

3. Such apprehensions were very prominent in the 18th and 19th centuries and some of the tales of Edgar Allan Poe, e.g. *The Cask of Amontillads* and *Premature Burial*, seemed only to increase such fears.

4. Moores, B., Clarke, G., Lewis, B. R., Mallick, N. P. 'Public Attitudes towards Kidney Transplantation', *Br. Med. J.* 1976, 629–31.

5. See Jennett, B. 'Brain Death', Editorial, *Br. J. Anaesthesia*, 1981, 53. ii. III5.
   Wilson, P. E., Cast, I., 'Donor Kidneys and restrictions on their supply', *Br. Med. J.* 1980, i.45.
   Jennett, B., 'Donor Supply in UK', *T. S. Annual Report*, London, HMSO. London 1981
   Kaufman, H. H., Hutchton, J. D., McBride, M. M., Beardsley, C. A., and Kahan, B. D., 'Kidney Donation; Needs and Possibilities', 5 *J. Neurosurg.*, 1979, 237.
   Walker, A. E., 'The Neurosurgeon's Responsibility for Organ Procurement'. 44 *J. Neurosurg.*, 1976, 1.

6. 'A. B. C. of Brain Stem Death: Reappraising Death', *Br. Med. J.* 285, 13 Nov, 1982, 1409.

7. Report of the Committee on Death Certification and Coroners (1971) Chairman, Mr Justice Brodick. HMSO.

See also Jennett, B., 'The donor doctor's dilemma: Observations on the recognition and management of brain death', *J. Med. Eth.* 1975, 1: 66.

8. Karen Ann Quinlan, the American woman (now aged 30, 20 March 1984), whose name became synonymous with the 'right to die' controversy, has spent eight years in an irreversible coma after mixing alcohol and drugs at a party. Her parents fought for the right to disconnect the life-support system that doctors believed was keeping her alive. The Quinlans won a year-old legal battle when the New Jersey Supreme Court ruling gave them permission to remove her from the respirator. Ann Quinlan however has continued to breathe on her own since the plug was pulled on her respirator.

9. Jennett, B., Plum, F., 'Persistent Vegetative State after Brain Damage: A Syndrome in search of a Name', *Lancet*, 1972, 1 April, 734–7.
See also 'Brain Death', Editorial, *Brit. J. of Anesth.* 1981, 53: II: 1111–9.
Jennett, B. Teasdale. G.
Davies, F. A., 'Management of Head Injuries', *Phil. USA.* 1981, 311f.

10. In *The Guiness Book of World Records.*, Ed. Norris McWhirter, 1981, 42, a case is recorded of Alaine Esposito who lapsed into coma following surgery on 6 August 1941 and died 25 November 1978, 37 years and 111 days later.

11. 'Brain Damage and Brain Death', *Lancet*, 1974, i: 341.

12. See also *Decisions about Life & Death: A Problem in Modern Medicine.* Board of Social Responsibility of the Church of England, C10. 1965, 52–3.
Papal Allocution of Pope Pius XII. Acta Apostolicae Sedis 49, 1957, 1033.
The Pope Speaks, iv. 398.
On Dying and Dying Well: Edwin Stevens Lecture, Royal Society of Medicine, 13 Dec, 1976. in *Sure Foundation*, Donald Coggan, Hodder & Stoughton, 1981. 90–106.
Dunstan, G., *The Artifice of Ethics*: The Moorfield Lecture, SCM Press, 1974, 89f.

13. *Br. Med. J.* 1980, 281: 1139–41. Jennett, B., Wilson, P., Gleavel, J. *Br. Med. J.* 1981, 282:533.
See also 'A Television verdict on Brain Death', Editorial, *Lancet*, 18 Oct. 1980.
'An appalling Panorama', Editorial, *Br. Med. J.* 1980, 281: 1028.
Calne, R. Y., Letter to Editor, *The Times*, London, 16 Oct 1980.
Johnson, R. W. G., Letter to Editor, *The Times*, London, 16 Oct 1980.
Pallis, C., 'Medicine and The Media,' *Br. Med. J.* 281: 1064.

14. Sweet, William H. 'Brain Death', Editorial, *New Eng. J. Med.* 1978, 24 August.

15. 'After the "definition of irreversible coma"', *New Eng. J. Med.* 1969, 281: 1070–1.

16. 'Brain Death: A clinical and pathological study': *J. Neurosurg.* 1971, 35.211.

17. 'Conference of Medical Royal Colleges and their Faculties in the UK: Diagnosis of Death', *Lancet*, 1976, ii: 1069. *Br. Med. J.* 1976, 2:1187–88.

18. 'Conference of Medical Royal Colleges and their Faculties in the UK: Diagnosis of Death', *Br. Med. J.*, 1979, 1: 332. *Lancet*, 1979, 1:261–2.

19. See Walker, A. E., 'The neurosurgeon's responsibility for organ procurement', *J. Neurosurg.*, 1976, 44:1.
    Mohanda, A., Cou, S. A., 'Brain Death: A clinical and pathological study', *J. Neurosurg.*, 1971, 35:211.
    'Brain Damage and Brain Death', *Lancet*, 1974: 1:341.
    'Brain Death:' *Br. Med. J.* : 1975: 1:356.
    MacGillivray, B., 'The diagnosis of cerebral death', art. in *Proceedings of the Tenth Congress of the European Dialysis and Transplant Association*: Ed. J. F. Moorhead, Pitman Medical, London, 1973.

20. See 'Brain Death': Letter from Professor J. G. Robson, Honorary Secretary, Conference of Medical Royal Colleges and their Faculties in the UK, *Br. Med. J.*, 1981, ii: 283: 505.

21. See Evans, D. W., Lum, L. C., 'Cardiac Transplantation', *Lancet*, 1980 1: 933–4.
    World Medicine, 14 May, 1983, Corresp. 'Understanding Brain Death'.
    Byrne, P. A., O'Reilly, S., Quay, P. M. 'Brain-death — an opposing viewpoint', *JAMA*, 1979, 242: 1985–90.

22. 'ABC of Brain Stem Death', *Br. Med. J.* 1982, 285: 20 November: 1487–8. See also Pallis, C. Commentary, 'Whole Brain Death Reconsidered: Physiological facts and Philosophy', *J. Med. Eth.* 1983, 9:32–7.
    Kennedy, I., *The Unmasking of Medicine: A searching look at Health Care Today*, Paladin Book, Granada, London. (Revised edition1983.) 201f.

23. See Skegg, P. D. G., 'The case for a statutory definition of death', *J. Med. Ethics*, 1976, 2:190–2.
    Skegg, P. D. G., 'Irreversible comatose individuals: Alive or Dead?', *Camb. Law J.*, 1974, 33:130–44.
    Skegg considers that many of the objections to a statutory definition of death are misplaced, and that such a statute would remove all doubts in the minds of both doctors and public as to whether a 'beating heart cadaver' was dead or alive for legal purposes.
    Cf. opposing viewpoints — e.g. Kennedy, I., 'The Definition of Death', *J. Med. Eth*, 1977, 3:5–6.
    Kennedy holds to the view that a more flexible code of practice which responds to medical opinion and which would be interpreted in good faith is to be preferred.
    Coggan, D., *On Dying and Dying Well: Sure Foundation*, Hodder & Stoughton, London, 1981, 104 — 'we would eschew the pursuit of legislation and let experience and wisdom decide.'

24. Walker, A. Earl, *Cerebral Death* (2nd Ed.), Urban & Schwarzenberg, Baltimore-Munich, 1981, p.177.

25. Pope Pius XII, Acta Apostolicae Sedis. 45, November 1957, 1027–33. Cf. Ramsey, P.: *The Patient as Person : Exploration in Medical Ethics*, Yale Univ. Press, New Haven and London, (6th ed.) 1975, 104 '. . . The determination of death is a medical matter . . . a theologian or moralist can offer only his reflections upon the meaning of respect for life and care of the dying'.

26. Haring, B., *Medical Ethics*, Notre Dame Ind. Fides Publ. Inc, pp 132–3. Haring writes that 'a general consensus has been reached that brain death is the end of the earthly history of a human person. With the destruction of the cerebral cortex, the material substratum of any spiritual activity is destroyed; man no longer has the possibility of realizing his personality in freedom and his human history comes to an end.'
The Jesuit priest, Fr John Mahoney, S. J. Heythrop College, London, sees the concept of brain death as 'a humane and helpful indication when decisions are required about whether or not to resuscitate or prolong intensive care procedures'. In such cases 'the presumption of the public at least is not that the patient has died but that the patient should now be allowed to die . . . whereas one might reasonably expect that cessation of brain activity would now be welcomed as an additional safeguard alongside heart death and lung death, on the contrary, brain death is proposed as an alternative criterion for pronouncing death even although the heart may continue for some time to beat spontaneously.'
Mahoney J., 'Transplants: The Definition of Death', *The Times*, 3 Feb 1975.
'Ethical Aspects of Donor Consent in Transplantation', *J. Med. Eth.* 1975, 1:67.

Chapter 4: Handicapped Infants — To Live or Let Die?

1. Freeman, J., *Practical Management of Meningomyelocele*, University Park Press, Baltimore, 1974, p. 16.

2. Potts, W. J., *The Surgeon and The Child*, Philadelphia, W. B. Saunders Co., 1959, p. 8.

3. For discussion of ethical issues involved in screening see Habgood, J., *A Working Faith*, Darton, Longman & Todd, 1980 pp. 177–85.
Fletcher, John, 'Moral and Ethical Problems of Pre-natal Diagnosis', 1975, *Clin. Genet.* 8: 251.

4. Medical Research Council working party on amniocentesis: 'An Assessment of the Hazards of Amniocentesis', *Br. J. Obstet. Gynaecol*, 1978, 85: Supple. 2:1–41.

5. Smithells, R. S., Sheppard, S., Schorach, C. J., Selle, M. J., Nevin, M., Horace, R., Read, A. P., Fielding, D. W., 'Possible Prevention of Neural Tube Defects by Periconceptual Vitamin Supplementation', *Lancet*, 1980 1:339–40.
   Laurence, K. M., James, N., Muller, M. H. *et al.*, 'Increased risk of recurrence of pregnancies complicated by fetal neural tube defect in mothers receiving poor diets, and the possible benefits of dietary counselling', *Br. Med. J.* 1980, 281:1592.
   Also: 'Double-blind randomized controlled trial of folate treatment before conception to prevent recurrence of neural-tube defect', *Br. Med. J.* 1981, 282:1509–11.

6. Harper, P., *Practical Genetic Counselling*, John Wright, Bristol, 1981.

7. WCC Study Encounter 1974, Vol. X : No. 1.

8. Lorber, J. 'Ethical problems in the management of myelomeningocele and hydrocephalus': The Milroy Lecture, *J. Roy. Coll. Phycns*, 1975, 10:1:47–60.

9. Lorber, J. 'Early results of selective treatment of spina bifida cyctica,' *Br. Med. J.* 1973, 27:201–4.

10. *Lancet*: 1975: 11 January: 85–8: Also reproduced in Habgood, J., *A Working Faith*, ibid: 161–176.

11. See Zachary, R. B., 'Life with Spina Bifida', *Br. Med. J.* 1977, 2: 1460. Zachary states: 'To leave a child without food is to kill it as deliberately and directly as if one was cutting its throat'.
    See also: Zachary, R. B., 'Ethics and Social Aspects of Treatment of Spina Bifida', *Lancet*, 1968, 2:274.
    de Lange, S. A., *Developmental Med. & Ch. Neurol.* 1974, 16: Suppl 32:27.

12. ATV: 'Jaywalking', Sunday, 22 February 1981: Thames TV Afternoon Plus, 15 January, and subsequently on BBC 2, Man Alive, 'A Loving Thing To Do', 26 February 1981.

13. 'Withholding Treatment in Infancy', *Br. Med. J.* 1: 925–6. Anon: 'Non-treatment of Defective Newborn Babies', *Lancet*, 1979, ii:1123–4. See also Duff, R. S., Campbell, A. G. M., 'Moral Ethical Dilemmas in the Special Care Nursery', 1973, *New Eng. J. Med.* 1973, 289:894.

14. The Linacre Centre, London, 1982: 5. See also p. 7. 'To say one is "letting a child die" is certainly a euphemism for killing when one is administering sedatives to a baby so that it shall be continuously sleepy, take little or no food and die within a few weeks. In such a case it is not the condition of spina bifida that causes the death of the child but the lack of nutrition.'

15. See Freeman, J. 'Is There a Right to Die?', *J. Pediatrics*, 1972, 80:904–5. Also 'The Shortsighted Treatment of Myelomeningocele', *J. Pediatrics*, 1974, 53:311–3.

16. 'Withholding treatment in infancy', Editorial: *Br. Med. J,* 1981, 282: 925–6.

17. Duff, R. J., Campbell, A. G. M., Authors response to Richard Sherlock, *J. Med Eth.,* 1979, 5:141.

18. Scorer, G. and Wing, A., Ed: *Decision Making in Medicine,* Edward Arnold, London, 1979.

19. *Prolongation of Life.* Paper 2: 'Is there a morally significant difference between killing and letting die?', Linacre Centre Papers, The Linacre Centre, London, 1978.
    See also Steinbock, Bonnie. Ed. *Killing and Letting Die,* Prentice Hall Inc. Englewood Cliffs N. J. 07632, 1980.

20. Ingelfinger, F. J., 'Bedside Ethics for the Hopeless Case', *New Eng. J. Med.* 1973, 289:885–90.

21. Walker, J. H., Thomas, M., Russell, I. T., *Developmental Med. Child Neurol.* 1971, 13: 462.
    See Allis, H. L., 'Parental involvement in the decision to treat spina bifida cystica', *Br. Med. J.* 1974, 2 March, 369–74.
    Also Campbell, A. G. M., Duff, R. S., 'Deciding the care of severely malformed or dying infants', *J. Med, Eth.,* 1979, 5:65–7.
    'Withholding treatment in infancy', Editorial, *Br. Med. J.,* 1981, 282:925–6.

22. Duff, R. S., Campbell, A. G. M., 'Moral and Ethical Dilemmas in the Special-Care Nursery', ibid., 1973, 289: 890–4.

23. See Kennedy, I., Letter, *The Times,* 7 January 1978, and *The Unmasking of Medicine: A Searching Look at Health Care Today,* Paladin, Granada, (Revised Ed.) 1983.
    Ramsey, P., *Ethics at the Edge of Life: Medical and Legal Intersections,* New Haven and London, Yale Univ. Press, 1978.
    McCormick, R. A., 'To Save or Let Die: The Dilemma of Modern Medicine', *J.A.M.A.,* 1974, 229: 175.
    'The Right to Live and the Right to Die', Editorial, *Br. Med. J.,* 29 August 1981, 569–70.

24. See Silverman, W. A., 'Mismatched Attitudes about Neonatal Death', *The Hastings Center Report.* 1981 Dec.,
    Also Stinson, R. and P., *The Long Dying of Baby Andrew,* Little Brown & Co., Boston and Toronto, 1983. A true story of what can happen when a baby becomes hopelessly entrapped in an intensive care unit where the machinery is more sophisticated than the code of law and ethics governing its use.
    Silverman, W. A., 'A Hospice Setting for Humane Neonatal Death', *Pediatrics,* 1982, 69:239–40.

25. Hare, E. H., Laurence, K. M., Payne, M. and Rawnsley, K., *Br. Med. J.,* 1966, ii:757.

See also 'Early Management of Handicapping Disorders', *IRMMH Reviews of Research and Practice*. 19. Ed. Oppe, T. E., and Woodford, F. P., Elsevier, *Excerpta Medica*, North Holland, 1976, 98.

26. Solnit, A. J., Stark, M., 'Mourning and the birth of a defective child,' *Psychoan. Stud. Child.* 1961, 16.

27. Lovell, A., 'When a Baby Dies', *New Society*, 14 April 1983, 65. The writer, himself a doctor, expresses his own reactions to his handicapped little daughter, Molly, who was on the Special Baby Unit operating table: — 'It was impossible not to want to hold her, feel her and hear human sounds instead of the electronic signs and blips and flickers which came to signify her life.'

28. See National Assoc. of Mental Health Working Party, (1971), 'The Birth of an Abnormal Child: Telling the Parents', *Lancet*, 2:1075. Darcy, E., 'Congenital Defects: Mothers' Reaction to First Information', *Br. Med. J.*, 1968, 3:796.
Drotar, D., Baskiewicz, A., Irvin, N., *et al.*, 'The Adaption of Parents to the Birth of an Infant with a Congenital Malformation: A Hypothetical Model', *Pediatrics*, 1975, 56:710.
John, N., 'Family reactions to the birth of a child with a congenital anomaly' *Br. Med. J.*, August 1971, 5:277.
Gath, A., 'The impact of an abnormal child upon the parents', *Brit J. Psychiat.* 1977, 130:405–10. Ann Gath matched 'thirty families with a newborn mongol baby with thirty families with a normal baby. Both groups were followed up for eighteen months to two years and interviewed six times. Few differences could be found in the mental or physical health of the two groups, but marital breakdown or severe marital disharmony was found in nine of the mongol families and in none of the controls . . . Despite their grief, the parents of almost half the mongol children in this study felt drawn closer together, and their marriage rather strengthened than weakened by their shared tragedy.'

29. Mitchell, R. G., 'Chronic handicap in childhood: Its implications for family and community', *Practitioner*, 1973, 211:763–8.
See two studies carried out in the Isle of Wight and Newcastle areas, Rutter, M., Tizard, J., Whitmore, K., *Education, Health and Behaviour*, Longmans, London, 1970.
Walker, J. H., Thomas, M., Russell, I. T., 'Spina Bifida and the Parents', *Develop. Med. Child Neurol.* 1971, 13: 456–61.

30. Zachary, R. B., 'Ethical and Social Aspects for treatment of Spina Bifida', *Lancet*, 1968, 2:274–7.

31. Fletcher, Joseph, *Humanhood: Essays in Biomedical Ethics*, Prometheus Books, New York, 1979, 7–19.
See also 'Indicators of Humanhood: A Tentative Profile of Man', *Hastings Center Report*, 1972, 5: 141.

32. Duff, R. J., Campbell, A. G. M., *J. Med. Eth.* 1979, 5:141.

33. McCormick, R. A. 'To Save or Let Die? The Dilemma of Modern Medicine', ibid 1974, 172–6.

34. Ramsey, Paul, *Ethics at Edges of Life*, ibid.

35. *Dying — considerations concerning the passage from life and death*, The Anglican Church of Canada Task Force on Human Life, The Anglican Book Centre, Toronto, Canada, 1980. It is emphasized that the Report is not a definitive statement setting forth official church positions.

36. See *Severely Abnormal Babies*, Interim statement of Church of England Board of Social Responsibility, CIO, 1 Feb. 1982.

37. 'The right to live and the right to die,' Editorial, *Br. Med. J.* ibid.

Chapter 5: Human Fertilization & Embryology

1. Snowden, R., Mitchell, G. D., *The Artificial Family*, Allen & Unwin, 1981, 55.

2. *Artificial Insemination*, RCOG, London, 1979.

3. See Brahams, D., 'In-Vitro Fertilization and Related Research', *Lancet*, 1983, September 24, 726–9.

4. (a) Report of a Commission appointed by His Grace the Archbishop of Canterbury, *Artificial Human Insemination*, SPCK, 1948.
   (b) Report of the Departmental Commission on Human Artificial Insemination, (Feversham) 1960, CMND 1105.
   (c) Peel Committee Report of the panel on Human Artificial Insemination, *Br. Med. J.*, 1973, 2: Suppl. Appendix V.3.
   (d) *Artificial Insemination*: Proceedings of the fourth study group of the RCOG, 1976.
   (e) *Choices in Childlessness*: The Report of a Working Party set up in July 1979 under the auspices of The Free Church Federal Council and The British Council of Churches, March 1982. 40.

5. *Artificial Insemination*: RCOG, ibid.

6. Evidence to the DHSS (Warnock) inquiry into human fertilization and embryology: Report by the Board of Social Responsibility, General Synod, GS Misc. 172:8.

7. 'Counselling for Access to Birth Records' *Adoption and Fostering*, 1983, 7:51.

8. See Dunstan, G., 'Ethical Aspects of Donor Insemination', *J. Med. Eth.* 1975, 1:42–44. Czyba, J. C., Manuel, C. 'Artificial Insemination with Donor Sperm. The French Experience,' *Scientific World*, 1981, 4, 21–24. Titmus, R. M., *The Gift Relationship*: From Human Blood to Social Policy, Allen & Unwin, London, 1973.

9. Curie-Cohen, M., Luttrell, L., Shapiro, S., 'Current practice of artificial insemination by donor in the United States', *N. Eng. J. Med.* 1979, 300:ii:585–90.

10. Quoted in Glass. D. V., Report of the Departmental Committee on Human Artificial Insemination, HMSO. 1960.

11. A lesbian woman in Sydney, Australia, gave birth to a baby 'conceived' by a 'do-it-yourself' artificial insemination kit, November 1981.

12. In three addresses Pope Pius XII uttered the basic magisterial pronouncements: (a) 'Address to the Fourth International Convention of Catholic Doctors', 29 September 1949: (b) 'Address to The Congress of the Italian Catholic Union of Midwives', 26 November 1951: (c) 'Address to the second world congress on fertility and sterility', 19 May 1956.

In condemning artificial insemination (AIH or AID) the following considerations were outlined:

1. Insemination outside the natural act of sexual intercourse 'would be the same as to convert the domestic hearth, which is the family sanctuary, into a mere biological laboratory.'
2. Artificial insemination would separate the unitive and procreative meaning of sexual intercourse, sundering by human action what is divinely intended to be inseparable.
3. Artificial insemination would entail immoral means for procuring sperm (masturbation).
4. Artificial insemination using donor sperm would violate the marriage covenant requiring that 'procreation of new life can only be the fruit of marriage.'

Pope Pius XII did grant exception to the prohibition of AIH in those situations in which the sperm was procured by a method other than 'acts contrary to nature', and where the act involved 'the use of certain artificial means designed only to facilitate the natural act or to enable that act, performed in a normal manner, to attain its end.'

13. *Choices in Childlessness*, ibid.

14. Davies, I., 'Close Encounters in a Test-Tube: Problems relating to artificial reproduction techniques', *Free Church Chronicle*, 1983, 1: XXVIII: 12–18. See *Law and Medical Ethics*: J. K. Mason, R. A. McCall Smith, Butterworths. London. 1983.

15. Edwards, R. G., 'Test-Tube Babies', *Nature*, 1981, 293: 253–6.

16. Edwards, R. G., Purdy, J., Ed. *Human Conception In Vitro*, London, 1981, 373.

17. Edwards, R. G., Purdy, J. Ed. ibid.

18. Fletcher, J., *The Ethics of Genetic Control: Ending reproductive roulette*,

Doubleday, Anchor Books, New York, 1974, 147–87.

19. Edwards, R. G., Horizon Lecture, BBC 2, 28 October 1983: 'Should the law be involved in the research and clinical aspects of human embryology? I do not think so, because our experience with other laws in the field gives us little confidence in believing that justice will or can be done . . . it would be far better to leave standards of practice primarily to the scientific and medical societies, especially those well versed in such affairs.'
See also 'Embryology needs rules, not new laws', Editorial, *Nature*, 1983, 302: 28 April: 735–6.

20. Report of the RCOG Ethics Committee on *In Vitro* Fertilization and Embryo Replacement or Transfer: 16.

21. See *In Vitro Fertilization Morality and Public Policy*: Evidence submitted to the government committee of inquiry into human fertilization and embryology (the Warnock Committee) by the Catholic Bishops' Committee on Bio-ethical Issues, on behalf of the Catholic Bishops of Great Britain, 2 March, 1983, 19–23.

22. Ramsey, P., *Fabricated Man: The Ethics of Genetic Control*, Yale University Press, USA, 1970, 39.

23. Taylor, G. R., *The Biological Bomb*, Thomas & Hudson, London, 1968, 179.

24. Edwards, R. G., 'Fertilization of Human Eggs *In Vitro*: Morals, Ethics and the Law'. *The Quarterly Review of Biology*, 1974, 49:3–26.

25. Report of the RCOG Ethics Committee on *In Vitro* Fertilization and Embryo Replacement or Transfer, ibid. ii.

26. Grobstein, C., 'Coming to terms with test-tube babies', *New Scientist*, 1982, 7 October, 14–17.

27. Trounson, A., Mohr, L., 'Human pregnancy following cryopreservation, thawing and transfer of an eight-cell embryo', *Nature*, 1983, 305: 20 October: 707–709.

28. Brahams, D., '*In Vitro* Fertilization and Related Research', ibid. 726–729.

29. Trounson, A., Conti, A., 'Research in human *in vitro* fertilization and embryo transfer', *Br. Med. J.* 1982, 285: 24 July: 244–8.

30. Harris, J., '*In Vitro* Fertilization: The Ethical Issues', *Phil. Quarterly* 1983, 33:132:226.

31. Grobstein, C., *New Scientist*, 1982, 7 October, 15.

32. *General Synod Report of Proceedings*, 1976, 7(3):695. See also Dunstan, G., 'The moral status of the human embryo:, A tradition recalled', *J. Med. Eth.* 1984. 1. 38–44.

33. Williamson, B., 'Gene Therapy', *Nature*, 298:416–18.

34. 'Research related to human fertilization and embryology': Statement by the Medical Research Council, *Br. Med. J.*, 1982, 285:1480. See other medical evidence submitted to the Warnock Committee by the Royal Society, Royal College of Obstetricians and Gynaecologists, British Medical Association, Royal College of General Practitioners.

35. *In Vitro Fertilization Morality and Public Policy*: Evidence submitted to the government committee of inquiry into human fertilization and embryology (the Warnock Committee) by the Catholic Bishops' Joint Committee on Bio-ethical Issues, on behalf of the Catholic Bishops of Great Britain, ibid. 7.

36. Fletcher, J., *The Ethics of Genetic Control*, ibid. 147–87.

37. Ramsey, P., *Fabricated Man*, ibid, 78, 108.
Habgood, J., *A Working Faith*, Darton, Longman & Todd, 1980, 155–160.

38. *Choices in Childlessness*, ibid.

39. Grobstein, C., *New Scientist*, 1982, ibid.
See *Human Procreation: Ethical aspects of the new techniques*. Report of a Working Party, Council for Science and Society, OUP, 1984.

Index of Proper Names

Aristotle, 190
Arthur, L., 111
Augustine, 190
Aquinas, 190

Baelz, P., 137, 162,
  165, 179, 193, 199
Balint, M., 38
Barnard, C., 47
Beecher, H. K., 39,
  94f
Bewick, M., 50, 52f,
  58f, 71, 106
Bishop of London,
  193
Brown, L., 168

Calne, R. Y., 62, 64,
  66, 74, 80
Campbell, A. G. M.,
  20, 119, 137, 145
Campbell, S., 113
Castle, K., 68, 76
Chalmers, I., 33, 133f
Chou, S. N., 95
Clark, B., 68
Clark, K., 101
Clayden, G., 129,
  132, 136, 146, 151
Cook, R., 124, 128,
  132, 147
Cory-Pearce, M., 70
Craft, I., 181, 184,
  186f, 199

Denham, M., 41f
Diamond, E., 151
Dominica, F., 138
Down, J. L., 110
Duff, R. S., 119, 137,
  145, 153

Dunstan, G. R., 59,
  88, 149
Dworking, G., 22f

Eckstein, H., 129, 133
Edwards, R. G., 168f,
  172f, 176, 188, 192,
  198, 201
Elwood, P., 29, 44f
Emery, A. E. H., 124,
  132
Enders, J., 25
English, T., 47, 63,
  68f, 73, 76
Evans, R., 121, 139

Farquharson, J., 111
Fletcher, J., 23, 129,
  145, 148f, 201

George, C., 10, 19, 41
Gillon, R., 18
Glover, J., 124, 126,
  130, 134, 147, 151f
Goodall, J., 121f, 136,
  153
Graham, R., 158
Gray, P., 120
Grobstein, C., 182,
  191, 202

Habgood, J., 149,
  194, 201
Hare, E. H., 140
Harper, P., 114
Harris, R., 158
Harrison, J. H., 47
Hibbard, B., 203
Huxley, A., 185

Ingelfinger, F. J., 15

Insley, J., 122, 131f,
  141

Jakobovits, I., 200
Jefferson, G., 10
Jenner, E., 9
Jennett, B., 50, 82,
  87f, 91f, 101f, 105,
  107
Jolly, H., 120, 123,
  139, 141f, 153

Kennedy, I., 23f, 61,
  126, 137, 148, 162,
  164, 180, 195
Knapp, M. S., 61

Lockwood, G., 33,
  152
Lockwood, M., 32,
  125, 130f, 147
Lorber, J., 116f, 119

Mahler, R., 36, 41
Mason, J. K., 82, 90,
  100, 104
Mawdsley, T., 136f
McCormick, R. A.,
  23, 145
McGeown, M., 75, 87
Merrill, J. P., 47
Mitchell, R. G., 143
Mohandas, A., 95
Morris, P., 49, 58, 64,
  71, 74, 87, 90, 100,
  105
Morrison, R., 177
Muller, H. J., 158
Murray, J. D., 47

O'Donovan, O., 178

Pallis, C., 85, 92, 102
Pappworth, M. H., 39, 44
Parsons, V., 49, 52, 56, 58, 65, 72, 75, 91, 99
Pearson, J., 36f, 111
Peel, J., 26, 160
Phipps, J., 9
Pius, Pope XII, 9, 89, 177
Plum, F., 88

Quinlan, K., 88

Ramsey, P., 14, 23, 146, 177, 201
Richens, A., 20, 34, 43
Ridler, M. A. C., 128
Robson, G., 99f

Ross, D., 47

Scanlon, J. W., 16, 40, 46
Sells, R. A., 54f, 58
Shumway, N., 47, 67, 74, 76
Silverman, W. A., 40, 134f, 138, 144
Singer, P., 147
Skegg, P. D. G., 22f
Slapak, M., 66, 87, 90
Starzl, T., 73f
Steptoe, P., 168f, 188
Stevas, St. J., 25
Sweet, W., 95

Tertullian, 190
Trounson, A., 172

Vere, D., 10f, 16, 18, 34, 41, 44, 46

Vitra, E., 68

Wade, O. L., 11, 19, 31, 38, 46
Walker, J. H., 143
Weil, W., 11, 44
Weller, T., 25
Wenham, G., 132
Whalan, D. J., 43
White, M., 124, 128, 135f, 150
Wilson, P. J., 49, 55, 71, 75, 81, 90, 99, 104
Withering, W., 9
Wolstenholme, G., 165
Wood, C. 172

Yacoub, M., 48, 68

Zachary, R. B., 143

Index of Subjects

Abdomen, 112f

Abnormalities, 164f, 188f, 215

Abortion, 2, 113, 174, 178, 188, 215

  Act, 113, 174f, 188

Act,

  Human Tissue, 52f

  Medicines, 27, 34f

Administrator, 54f

Adoption, 155f, 160, 184

Adultery, 167f

Alpha-feto-protein, 112f

Amniocentesis, 112f, 172f, 216

Anaestheticists, Congress of, 89

Analgesics, 117, 124, 216

Anencephaly, 111, 124

Animals, laboratory, 34

Animus, 190

Antibiotic, 88f, 110, 117, 216

Anxiety, 18

Artificial Insemination, AIH, 155f

  AID, 155f, 165f, 186, 215f.

  ethical concerns, 162f, 165, 166f, 186, 215f

  legal and social concerns, 159f, 162f, 165f, 186, 215f

Aspirin, 30

Assembly, General, of Church of Scotland, 59

Assault, 14

Assessment, Programme of, 69f, 76f, 140f

Association, British Medical, 16, 39, 182

  Paediatric, 22f

Banks, Sperm, 157f, 215

Barbiturates, 86f

Benefits, 15, 17, 22, 34

Beta-blockers, 30

Birth Certificate, 163f

Blastocyst, 195f, 216

Brain damage, 68, 81f, 89, 96

Brain death, 2, 81f, 86f, 96, 101f, 214f

  structure of, 92f

Brain-stem, 82f, 86, 95, 99, 101f

Burial, Premature, 84

Cadaver, 57f, 63f, 85f, 216

Cancer, 18, 49, 198

Care, Nursing, 19, 86, 90, 121, 135

Catheter, 96, 156, 216

Cells, 175f, 189f, 198f

Censuses, Office of Population, 155

Cerebrum, 93, 146, 148

Chaplains, Hospital, 1f, 120f

Chemotherapy, 16, 18

Chorea, Huntingdon's, 155f, 164f

Choroid plexus, 174

Chromosomes, 110f, 169f, 197f, 216

Church, Anglican, 106f, 167f, 178

  Free, 161f

  Roman Catholic, 106f, 167f, 178, 190

Circular, Guidance, 56f, 100f

Cloning, 200f, 216

Code, Minnesota, 95f

Colleges, Royal, Criteria, 83f, 92, 96f, 214f

Coma,
Drug-induced, 86f
Irreversible, 81, 95

Comatose, 96, 216f

Commission, 123f

Committee, Brodick, 86f
Ethical, 18, 22, 32, 39f, 41f, 186
Feversham, 160f
Safety of Medicines, 34f
Scientific Advisory, 41
Warnock, 185f, 200f

Compassion, 124

Compensation, 35, 37

Computers, 35, 62

Conception, 115f, 167f, 190f

Conceptus, 217

Conference, Lambeth, 167f

Confidentiality, 35

Consent, Informed, 12f, 14f, 21, 23, 34, 44, 55, 89, 91, 213f

Consciousness, 81, 92, 147

Contraception, 155f, 190f, 198f

Contracting, In, 53f, 56f
Out, 53f, 56f

Control Group, 29, 31

Co-ordinators, 51

Cornea, 96

Corpse, 84f

Cortex, 82, 88, 95f, 216

Council, Medical Research, 13, 21, 40, 47, 174, 198, 200

Counselling, Genetic, 114, 163, 180
Non-directive, 114f

Counsellor, 120, 163, 180

Court, Ward of, 111f

Cryostorage, 171f, 180f, 182f, 186, 189

Cyclosporin A, 63f, 67, 73, 75

Cystic Fibrosis, 197f

Death, cerebral, 82f, 100
clinical, 82f, 100
legal definition, 85, 104f
moment of, 84f, 89

Decapitation, 106

Decision-making, 41, 61, 119, 128f, 130f, 137f, 214f

Defect, Congenital, 108

Department of Health and Social Security, 54, 62

Diabetic, 74

Diagnosis, 17, 28, 97, 100, 217

Dialyser, 61f, 75

Dialysis, Continuous Ambulatory Peritoneal (CAP), 62f

Directors, Spiritual, 120f

Disorder, Inherited, 156f, 164f

Divorce, 178

Donation, Egg, 186f

Donation, Organ, 48f, 50, 53f, 70

Donor Cards, 51f, 59, 84, 92

Donors, Cadaver, 67f
potential, 57, 62
related, 65f
unrelated, 66f

Down's Syndrome, 110f, 124, 143, 152, 215

Drugs,
depressant, 86, 96
fertility, 154f
relaxant, 96

Dystrophy, Muscular, 197f

Ectogenesis, 175f, 217

Egg,
moral status, 192f
replacement, 181f
spare, 181f
transfer, 181f

Electro-encephalogran (EEG), 87, 94, 96f, 99, 217

Encephalitis, 43, 116f

Embryology, 2, 154f, 170, 188, 202, 217

Embryo, 170f, 176f, 180f, 182f, 187f, 189f

Ensoulment, 190f

Ethic, Christian, 42f, 44, 56, 59, 74, 78f, 89, 91f, 104f, 108, 118, 149, 116f, 190f, 201f, 214f

Ethicist, 2, 146, 149

Ethics, Handbook of Medical, 16, 66, 13, 138f

medical, 1f, 18, 21, 29, 34f, 44f, 56f, 78f, 89, 104f, 145f, 149, 156, 166f, 200f, 214f

Eugenics, 158

Euthanasia, 2, 91, 118

Experimentation,
Animal, 27, 43

children, 20f

embryonic, 189f, 195f

human, 2, 9f, 15, 204f, 213f

non-therapeutic, 13f, 20, 22f, 25, 208f

Failure, Renal, 60f

Family, Impact on, 139f

Fees, 165f

Fertilization, Ethical Concerns, 185f, 195f, 215f

human, 2, 154f, 169f, 191, 215f

in vitro, 168f, 195f, 215f

legal and social concerns, 176f, 195f, 215f

Fetus, 25, 146f, 174f, 188f, 217

Finance, 70f

Fluid, Seminal, 169f, 179f

Follicles, 169f, 217

Genes, 175, 197, 215, 217

Genetic, Engineering, 197f

manipulation, 175

therapy, 176f

Gestation, 26, 217

Grafting, Kidney, 61f

Guardians, 17, 22

Guidelines, Ethical, 214f

medical, 61, 64, 116f, 134, 145

Guilt, 138f, 143f

Haemodialysis, 60f, 82

Haemophilia, 173, 197

Haemorrhage, 67f, 82f, 217

Handicapped, Mentally, 17, 21, 91, 144, 146, 150f

Harvard Criteria, 94f

Heart, Artificial, 68, 73

beat, 67f, 81f, 84f, 98, 103

Helen House, 40, 144

Helsinki, Declaration of, 9, 13f, 18, 28, 46

Hindus, 78

Hip-replacement, 70

Homeostasis, 81

Hospices, 144f

Humanness, 145f, 193, 200

Hybrids, Human-Animal, 176f

Hydrocephalus, 110, 118, 142

Hypothermia, 86, 217

Hypothesis, Null, 29

Illegitimacy, 164

Immunology, 47, 63

Implantation, 170f, 189f, 190f, 194f

Incest, 166f, 184

Incubator, 169

Indicators, 145f

Infants, Handicapped, 2, 108f, 144, 146, 150f

new-born, 108f, 144, 146

Infanticide, 123f

Infarction, Myocardial, 30, 48, 54, 83, 218

Infection, 20, 110, 117

Insemination, 159f, 167f

Intercourse, Sexual, 159f, 168f, 178f, 189, 215

Intoxication, Drug, 86f
Intra-uterine device, 190
Investigator, 15f, 19f, 28, 31, 35, 38, 45, 209
Irreversibility, 83f
Iso-electric, 94f, 100

Jews, Orthodox, 78, 106
Journal, British Medical, 118f, 150

Lancet, The, 89
Laparoscope, 169
Law Society, 159f, 166f
Laws, Code of, 106
Life,
    prolongation of, 89f
    quality of, 108, 129, 150f
    sanctity of, 108, 128, 149, 150f, 199, 201f, 214f
Literature, Rabbinical, 106

Machines, Dialysis, 61f, 75
Man, dignity of, 14f, 35, 38
Masturbation, 156f
Means,
    extra-ordinary, 89
    ordinary, 89
Measures, Heroic, 89f
Medulla Oblongata, 93
Memory, 81
Meningitis, 110
Meningomyelocele, 108f
Mid-brain, 93
Miscarriage, 171f, 188f, 190f, 217
Mismatch, 137f
Mongolism, 110f, 124
Mourning, 140f
Muslims, 78

Negligence, 36
Neonates, 108f, 218
Nephrologist, 57, 218

Neural Tube Defect, (NTD), 112f, 218
Neurologists, 94, 218
Neurosurgeons, 94, 99
Next of kin, 49, 85, 90
Nuclei, 218
Nuremberg Code, 12
Nurses, 19, 86, 90, 96, 121, 135

Obstetricians and Gynaecologists, Royal College of, 160f, 176f, 181f, 188, 191f, 200
Omission, 123f
Organization, World Health, 46, 175
Organism, 101f, 146f, 191f
Organogenesis, 195f
Ovary, 156, 185f, 218
Ovulation, 156, 172
Ovum, 170f, 172, 186, 194
Oxygen, 102f, 117

Paediatrician, 108, 116, 135, 137f, 147f, 218
Panorama (BBC), 64f, 91f
Parents, 21, 24, 115f, 130
Payment, Volunteers, 31f, 34, 36
Peers, 34, 137
Perjury, 159f
Person, 145f
Personhood, 145f, 214f
Philosophers, 32, 129, 146, 149, 151
Physicians, Royal College of, 39
Physiotherapy, 28, 218
Placebo, 10, 29f, 32f, 218
Placenta, 174f, 191, 218
Pneumonia, 88
Polls, Gallup, 50f
    opinion, 48
Pontine Levels of brain, 92f
Practitioners, General, 40
    Royal College of, 40, 181

Pregnancy, 31, 114, 129, 134,
    154f, 165f, 170f
Priests, Parish, 2, 120
Procedure, Screening, 112f
Procreation, 117f
Profession, Medical, 19
Professionalism, 11f, 19
Prognosis, 17, 122, 218
Protocol, 25, 29
Putrefaction, 102f

Quickening, 190f

Radio-isotopes, 42
Radiotherapy, 28, 219
Recombination, 175f
Reflexes, 96
Rehabilitation, 128
Rejection, 47f
Relationships, 1, 145, 149
    Doctor-Patient, 14, 16f, 37f
Relatives, 21, 48f, 52, 55, 85, 90,
    100, 104, 119, 131f
Report, Ad Hoc Committee, 88,
    94f
    Harvard, 94f
    Board of Social
        Responsibility, 161f
    Church of Canada, 146
    Clarke, 61
    Free Church Federal Council
        & British Council of
        Churches, 161f
    Maclennan, 56f
    Pearson, 36f
    Peel, 160f
Research, 13f, 23f, 27, 35f, 39,
    173f, 196f, 199
    clinical, 13, 27
    biomedical, 13, 173f, 195f, 199
Resources, Financial, 70f
Respirators, 67, 73, 82f, 85, 87,
    89, 96f, 103f, 142
Responsibility, 43, 61

Resuscitation, 83, 117, 219
Rights, Individual, 29, 32f, 43
    of Society, 32f, 43, 64
Risks, 13, 15, 17, 24

Scan, Ultra-sound, 112f
Schools, Medical, 12, 46
Sedation, 117, 119, 219
Self awareness, 147f
    sacrifice, 34
Semen, 157, 165f, 169f
    frozen, 165f
Sentience, 90, 194f
Sex selection, 185f
Siblings, 120
Society, British Transplant, 59f
Sperm, 157f, 168f, 172, 179, 186,
    215, 219
Spermatozoa, 172, 179, 186, 215
Spina bifida, 108f, 140, 143, 197
Statistician, 42
Sterilization, 156
Still-born, 219
Stimuli, 86
Stress, 18f
Students, Medical, 12, 31, 46
Subject, 19, 35f
Surrogate motherhood, 171f,
    183f
Synod, General, 193

Temperature, 97
Test-tube babies, 168f, 176f, 199
Testes, 168
Theologian, 14, 94, 199
Therapeutics, 46
Tissue-typing, 61f
Totality, Principle of, 78
Toxicology, 29, 34, 87
Transplantation,
    Heart, 47f, 57, 67f, 71, 75,
        213f
    Heart/Lung, 48, 74, 213f
    Kidney, 47f, 54, 57, 61f, 64,

71, 213f
Liver, 48, 57, 73, 213f
Organ 2, 47f, 57f, 98f, 201, 213f
Pancreas, 74
Trauma, Cerebral, 88, 98
Treatment, Selective, 117f, 123f
Trials,
　clinical, 27f, 29, 32, 34
　double-blind, 29f
　psychiatric, 18
　randomized, 28f, 30, 33
Twinning, 191f

Unconscious, 84, 86, 89
Units,
　intensive care 2f, 82f, 84
　renal, 61
　special baby care, 175f
Universities, 46
Urethra, 155f

Uterus, 112, 190, 219

Vaccination, 43
Vaccines, 28, 219
Vasectomy, 158
Vegetative state, 87f
Ventilation, Artificial, 67, 73, 82f, 85, 89, 96f, 103f, 142
Viability, 26, 219
Visitor, Health, 128f
Vitamins, 114
Volunteers, 24, 31, 34, 44, 59, 164

Weight, Low birth, 108f
Witness, Jehovah, 79
Worker, Social, 137
Womb Leasing, 171f, 183, 186
World Council of Churches 115

Zygote, 191f, 219